# A Life with More Ups than Downs

# A Life with More Ups than Downs

*Albert Louis Elias*

iUniverse, Inc.

New York  Lincoln  Shanghai

# A Life with More Ups than Downs

iUniverse books may be ordered through booksellers or by contacting:

iUniverse
2021 Pine Lake Road, Suite 100
Lincoln, NE 68512
www.iuniverse.com
1-800-Authors (1-800-288-4677)

ISBN-13: 978-0-595-37213-3 (pbk)
ISBN-13: 978-0-595-81611-8 (ebk)
ISBN-10: 0-595-37213-9 (pbk)
ISBN-10: 0-595-81611-8 (ebk)

Printed in the United States of America

*"I do the very best I know how—the very best I can; and I mean to keep doing so until the end. If the end brings me out all right, what is said against me won't amount to anything. If the end brings me out wrong, ten angels swearing I was right would make no difference."*

—Abe Lincoln

# Contents

Preface . . . . . . . . . . . . . . . . . . . . . . . . . . . . . . . . . . . . . . . . . . xi

CHAPTER 1    The Early Years, 1946–1965 . . . . . . . . . . . . . . . . . . . 1

CHAPTER 2    The College Years, 1966–1969 . . . . . . . . . . . . . . . . 59

CHAPTER 3    Work, 1969–1976. . . . . . . . . . . . . . . . . . . . . . . . . . . 69

CHAPTER 4    Boston, November 1976–November 1977 . . . . . . . . 91

CHAPTER 5    Scarsdale, November 1977–June 1997 . . . . . . . . . . 94

CHAPTER 6    The Present, June 1997 . . . . . . . . . . . . . . . . . . . . . 104

# *Acknowledgements*

To Louise Albert for all her help and support throughout this project

# *Preface*

A journey of celebration. My life began on November 9, 1946. As I grew, I could not walk or talk well, as a result of cerebral palsy, but that has not stopped me from living life to its fullest. I have made a life for myself by simply celebrating what's there and doing the best I can. I have taken great comfort in reading some of our great thinkers, people like Socrates, Lincoln, Nietzsche, Gandhi, and Viktor Frankl, the Viennese psychiatrist who survived his years in the concentration camps by using his imagination to build an inner life that sustained him through his ordeals.

Through my reading of these great thinkers, I have gained both the comfort and strength to carry on.

I have also gained knowledge through a book with a provocative title, *If You Meet the Buddha on the Road, Kill Him*. I always have learned to trust my own knowledge and beliefs rather than the so-called experts.

When I was eighteen, my parents took me to an unusual orthopedic specialist. Instead of sitting behind his desk, this doctor came over to me and said, "These people sitting next to you know a lot more about you and what's best for you than I do. Be grateful that your parents have never allowed anyone to hurt you.

"You're obviously doing well," he continued, "so just keep on doing whatever it is you're doing. It seems to be working."

The first fifty-eight years have been exciting and I hope whatever time is remaining is equally rewarding.

Life can be exciting when you learn to look beyond the bad things that have happened in your life and allow yourself to enjoy the everyday good things that are all around us.

If this philosophy is followed, then each and every one of us can say that we had a life with more ups than downs.

# 1

# *The Early Years*

✦

## *1946–1965*

I was born on November 9, 1946, with a birth injury that the doctors diagnosed as cerebral palsy. I didn't walk until I was six, and then with great difficulty. From the age of two I slept in a splint. The splint had a pair of shoes attached to an iron bar in an effort to keep my legs apart. I then went on to short leg braces. I also have trouble with my eyes. To this day, I can't use both eyes together.

Shortly after I was born, the doctor recommended I be sent to Haverstraw, a rehabilitation center. My parents had such faith in the doctor that they were going to send me there sight unseen. But luckily my parents visited the place first with a neighbor and were shocked at what they saw. This marked the turning point in my life. Who can say what would have happened to me had my parents sent me to that rehab center.

My parents at that point decided to bring me up themselves and treat me like any normal child. When they took me with them to visit their friends, they would set me down on the floor and I'd take off and explore the new territory.

When I finally started to walk, it was in large part thanks to my maternal grandfather. He was an idealistic lawyer and because it was so important to him to be able to help people who needed legal advice even if they had no money, he often accepted payment in the form of barter.

One such barter client was an unemployed engineer. During one of their meetings, my grandfather told him how fascinated I'd become with the lights on the switchboard in their apartment lobby. I also loved to watch the light on the rather complicated telephone system my grandfather had rigged up in his apartment, with lights for each phone line, one red and one green. He asked the engineer to build a standing table with buttons that could light up pictures of clowns, cowboys and animals—the kinds of things a little boy would like to see. "If we put them on a table," he said, "so that Albert would have to stand to press the buttons to make the pictures light up, I'll bet he would try even harder to stand—and then eventually, he'll be able to walk."

Back in the late 40s this was a novel idea. It was before computers and video games. A kid today wouldn't find this table very magical, but I surely did, and still do when I think back to those early days.

Anyway, the engineer designed the table as his payment to my grandfather, and after many weeks of trying—and falling—and trying again, I finally was able to pull myself up and push the buttons.

A few months later, with the aid of my father, I started walking, though with a spastic gait, and have been doing so unaided until I turned fifty. Nowadays I still walk, maybe not as far, but I do it with the aid of a walker.

Floors have an unfortunate tendency to merge into stairs. When that happened when I was a kid, there was only one thing to do. One of my earliest memories was going down the stairs head first. People gasped when they saw this, and my parents lost a few so-called friends who thought that my parents were out of their minds to let me do this. When I got older and was able to walk, I still had trouble with stairs, but learned to go down them in a different way.

I remember visiting my brother many years later and coming downstairs from the second floor guest room: I did what I had to do. And soon I heard my three-year-old niece call to her mother, "Mommie, Mommie! Uncle Albert is going down the stairs on his bum," her word for backside. And to this day, whenever she and I come to a set of stairs, she turns to me and says, "Uncle Albert, just go down on your bum."

Unfortunately, not everyone is as accepting (and even admiring) as my niece of my unorthodox ways of solving my problems, so I have often been subjected to stares or rude comments. This has upset me, but not stopped me. Over the years I've lost a few battles, but I've still remained in the fight. Sometimes I've had to retreat and go after a goal with a new and better strategy.

This was certainly the case when it came time for me to enter kindergarten. The local school would not accept me. Though I was six years old, I still got around by crawling. Something in the local fire or school laws stated that people like me could only be home-schooled. That was the last thing my parents and I wanted. It was time to move on.

My parents found a very practical house in Upper Brookville, Long Island to move to. It was all on one floor. The local public school only had about one hundred kids from kindergarten through eighth grade and was more than happy to enroll me. The small physical campus suited me fine.

I remember being met at the school's front door by my teacher, Mrs. Ethel Frye. She had red hair and was only about five feet tall. (Later, when I was older and was just about fully grown and our families became good friends, when I stood up straight, we were about the same height.) She had a warm smile that made me feel comfortable and soon I was off and crawling!

I don't remember the other children's reactions to seeing me crawling around the classroom, but I do know I wasn't stopped from doing about any activity I set out to do. And I remember Mrs. Frye introducing me to the other children, or to grown-ups who would come into her classroom, as "Albert—he's the one on his knees."

I might have been on my knees, but I wasn't stuck that way. I crawled around so well that after a while most of the other kids got used to me and didn't seem to be frightened of me. Sometimes one or another child would call me a name, as though they were giving me a label, but listening to the advice of my parents, I tried not to let it bother me, because eventually I knew it was just a description of my physical appearance.

Mrs. Frye and her husband became lifelong family friends and there was no favor too big that they were unwilling to perform. Pick up my father at the airport at 6:00 A.M.? Sure, why not. I was certainly lucky to have had Mrs. Frye as my first teacher.

I was still "on my knees" when spring arrived that first year in school. With it came the warmer weather, and everyone longing to be playing out of doors. People seemed to come alive when the flowers started to bloom, and I was no exception.

I can still remember one particular day. The temperature was unusually warm for April, and Mrs. Frye announced to the class that because it was so nice outside, she would extend the recess period an extra half hour, "starting right now." There were shouts of joy as we all rushed to the door, each one wanting to be the first one on the playground.

I started crawling my way to the door, and although I moved quite fast on all fours, I was no match for the rest of the class who could move even faster on their two legs. By the time I had reached the door, I found that it was closed and I was alone in that huge classroom.

What was I going to do?

I started screaming, "Mrs. Frye! Mrs. Frye!" But my voice was not heard. Then I tried banging on the walls with my one good hand. That too went unnoticed.

I was all alone and feeling miserably frustrated. If only I could walk and run like the other kids. I knew they must be having fun out there. But just when I was at my lowest ebb and seeing no solution to my problem, an image of my grandfather entered my head. He was right next to the standing table, pointing to the pictures waiting to be lit up. He was showing me how to push the buttons to light up the clown and the cowboy. "Remember, Albert, I've seen you do it. I know you can pull yourself up again and touch the buttons. Don't give up now."

I wanted to say, "Yes, I did stand and press the buttons. But that was when you were right next to me. It's too hard to do it now without you. I can't do it alone." And then I looked at the door handle and saw my grandfather's hand turning it. The door opened and revealed the bright sunshine outside and the children playing on the grass. The door closed and my grandfather vanished.

I sat there looking at the handle on the door. "I can't open the door," I said to myself. "I just can't." But then I thought, Grandpa didn't let me quit, and he wouldn't want me to quit now. I kept hearing his voice echoing in my ear, "Try, Albert. Grandma and I know you can do it. Grandma and I know you can do it."

The words kept repeating until I could stand it no longer. Suddenly I began to crawl closer to the wall; reaching up to the windowsill with my good hand, I pulled myself up. For the first time in school, and on my own, I was standing. The view of the other kids running and playing made me want to be out there with them more than anything I could imagine. I knew now that I could manage to open the door, but I didn't want to go out there crawling. I wanted desperately to walk.

Again my eyes focused on the door leading to the playground and I saw Grandpa beckoning me to walk over to him. The door was open. I felt the warmth of the spring sun. I wanted to walk out there and play with my friends. I knew I had to try.

Holding on to the window ledge, this time with both hands, I slowly moved toward the door. My legs ached with pain, but by now I had gotten used to that feeling from all time I had worked on learning to walk with my father and my grandfather. Then, they had always held on to me. Now I was alone and frightened. Could I do it by myself? I felt my eyes fill up with tears, but I knew I couldn't give up, not only for my father and grandfather's sake, but for my own sake. And right then and there, I decided I would never be a quitter. I might lose a round or two, but I would never give up playing the game. And with that, I continued moving slowly until I reached the door.

When I got there, I turned the handle with my left hand and, pushing against it, I held on to the door frame and stood looking at everyone playing outside.

Grandpa was nowhere to be seen, but I heard applause ringing through my head, and knew my whole family was there with me.

Now what was I going to do? The idea of getting down on my knees and crawling was something I refused to do. So, by taking small, shuffling steps, I began to walk slowly without holding on to anything. But soon I fell. This time, however, I didn't let the fall upset me, and seeing a bench nearby, I slowly crawled over to it. I was now confident that if I held on to something I would be able to pull myself up. And that's exactly what happened. I then continued my quest to meet my classmates on the playground.

My legs were wobbly as I started across the ball field, but I held my hands out to the side and thought of the picture of the tightrope walker in the book that Mrs. Frye had read to us about the circus. It seemed to work, for I didn't lose my balance as I made my way to the middle of the playground to be with my friend, Paul, who was just about to catch a ball. He was playing catch with Bill.

"Paul," I said, "can I play, too?"

"Sure," Paul said, turning around to see where the voice came from. All at once his mouth and eyes were wide open, but nothing was coming out. Finally, he yelled, "Mrs. Frye! Mrs. Frye! Look! Albert is walking!"

Mrs. Frye, and everyone else, came running toward us to witness the "miracle" with their own eyes.

I couldn't play catch very well with the boys, but they were very nice to me when I kept dropping the ball. My big triumph came when I walked back to the classroom on my own.

I remained on my feet for the rest of the day and for the remainder of the school year. No more would Mrs. Frye refer to me, however kindly, as "Albert, the one on his knees." For now I was standing. Maybe my knees weren't as straight as the other kids', but I was standing and walking.

I don't know what my classmates thought of my new achievements, but it didn't really matter. The only thing I know was that my parents told me that Mrs. Frye had called that evening to say that I was standing and playing ball, and how exciting it was for the other children to see me walk.

The year ended with Mrs. Frye kissing us all good-bye. It was the first time I was kissed by somebody other than my mother. I felt rather nice. She also said, "Albert, keep up your good work. I expect to hear glowing reports from Miss Mac about you."

Miss Mac would have to wait until the fall, because starting in the end of June, I was beginning a new adventure—summer camp!

At North Shore Day Camp, I was again the only disabled person, but from the first day I was made to feel right at home. There was a special camp T-shirt and cap, both with the camp logo. All of the kids wore shorts, but I was always in long pants. I guess even then I was conscious of the appearance of my spastic legs, and although I must have looked the same whether dressed in long or short pants, I felt more secure when my legs were totally covered.

By the time camp started, I was only having occasional falls when I walked. Somehow, the occasional falls didn't stop me from playing baseball, however badly, or learning to shoot a bow and arrow with the help of another camper. The best thing, though, that I learned at North Shore Day Camp was how to swim, thanks to Mr. Thomas. Swimming really helped to relax my muscles, and by the time I left camp, I was one of the best swimmers.

When you swim, you use different muscles from those you use when you're walking. I became especially adept at swimming on my back. My whole body seemed to move freely through any depth of water. And my side stroke was good enough for me to swim in a team relay race. I even did a fairly good front dive, although I had to be helped onto the diving board and out almost to the edge before I could be left on my own to dive. I don't know what the other kids thought about helping me. Maybe they felt very grown-up having to take on the responsibility of helping to look after me. Whatever they felt, I know I was having fun.

Shop and science were also filled with challenges. I had a buddy in those activities and together we made Indian ashtrays and collected butterflies. All in all, camp was a wonderful experience, and when it ended, I couldn't wait till the next summer to do more swimming, and maybe to play some real baseball.

Fall came, and I started first grade with Miss Mac. From the start, she was just as understanding and helpful as Mrs. Frye had been. But it soon became clear to everyone that I was going to have a lot of problems writing with my one good hand. So it was suggested that I learn to use a manual typewriter in the classroom. My parents bought me a typewriter, and before long I was all set up. My desk was moved so that I was next to Miss Mac's desk, and from then until the seventh grade, I always had a desk next to the teacher.

The typewriter proved to be just the thing to help me communicate with other people, because, unfortunately, another side effect of my cerebral palsy was inability to speak without a severe stutter. This speech problem persisted until my senior year in high school. In the meantime, people either had to wait for me to type something, or take the time to make sense of my stuttering speech. It was a hard time for me, and there were many times back then when I found myself all alone.

For me, only seven, just beginning to walk and now having to learn to type, I was often left with a feeling of being very different, and of being rejected. But somehow I managed to deal with it, as I was so pleased to be learning so many new skills. One of them was to try not to pay attention to what the outside world thought of me. It wasn't until I was at college, and on my own, that the painful feelings of isolation would sometimes be overwhelming.

But back to first grade. Miss Mac lived with her parents on a horse farm. One spring day our class took a field trip out to the farm and it was there that I had my first experience, not only sitting on a horse, but actually riding it!

Earlier that year, I was introduced to Gilbert and Sullivan's operetta, *The Pirates of Penzance*. This began a lifelong love affair with light vocal music. But more of that later. For now, let me tell you about my friendship with Chris, a seventh grader whom I met when I attended a rehearsal of *The Pirates*. Because of my disability, I was befriended by several older kids, and it was because of them that I was allowed to watch rehearsals of the operetta, and I soon became a kind of mascot for them. Before long, I had learned all the words that Chris sang in his role as the Modern Major General. Luckily for Chris, I sang in a monotone, so Chris didn't have to worry.

At the end of the production, Chris rewarded me for my enthusiasm with a gift of his costume. I just loved the red jacket with its bright gold epaulets. I wore the costume to Miss Mac's farm and I was lifted up onto a big white horse by her father. I sat up straight and tall and felt that I was the very model of a Modern Major General.

I continued to love music, and soon my parents bought me a record player. With my dog Muffin, I would sit for hours listening to everything from classical music to show tunes from such shows as *My Fair Lady*, *Kiss Me, Kate*, and *South Pacific*.

Music stimulated new sensations in me, and for some reason, I found myself making up little adventure stories to go with the songs. There was a never-ending stream of ideas that were flowing through my head. When I listened to my records, I didn't feel alone, but was somehow connected to other people through my imagination.

My imagination has served me well throughout my life. Even when I seem to be at my lowest ebb, a song will mysteriously play in my head and I will be off on a brand new adventure and my feelings of inadequacy will have vanished. In its place will be a new insight into what it was that was making me so upset. Music provides me with a wonderful way of helping myself to climb out of the deepest feelings of despair.

My schooling continued, but in the seventh grade I had to say good-bye to my typewriter in the classroom. Mr. Johnson, my teacher, wanted me to write in class by hand, and he said he would somehow manage to decipher my attempt at printing.

Mr. Larry Johnson was a man in his late twenties who did his best to stimulate his classes, not only intellectually, but emotionally as well. Each night we were assigned to watch the evening news and to write up some item that was of special interest to us. I found myself drawn to any news having to do with international relations. Soon I knew a lot about Soviet-American conflicts, Cuban-American issues, and the split between Russia and China. I couldn't wait till dinner ended each evening so that I could watch the news and pick out my next writing assignment. Besides assigning us to watch the news, he had us all subscribe to the *New York Herald Tribune*. I felt very grown-up walking into the classroom each morning and finding the newspaper lying on my desk. My family had the *New York Times* delivered to our home, but my father always took it to work. Now I had a newspaper of my own and could read it whenever I wanted to, and I compared the newspaper coverage to that of the evening TV news.

Mr. Johnson never gave us homework on the weekends. However, he did offer extra credit for those of us who wanted to write at that time. We could choose any subject. And so many a weekend you would find me at the typewriter writing a short piece about Abraham Lincoln or about one of the other great figures I spoke about in my introduction. My parents were pleased that I took on this extra work. I guess it not only reinforced their own convictions that they had done the right thing by sending me to a regular school, but more importantly, they knew I was gaining a skill that I would use for the rest of my life. I had learned to amuse myself and to become my own best friend. This was really an important achievement because already I could see that I would not be included in many of my peers' activities. Being self-reliant was to become an essential skill for me.

Despite the above, both my parents and Mr. Johnson thought I would benefit from the help of a tutor in math and general schoolwork as well. My parents contacted the people at Hunter College to help find such a person for me and all my special needs. Both my parents and I were very surprised when the tutor they sent, Richard Switzer, was an adult with cerebral palsy. He was great for me, for not only did he help me with my schoolwork but with various social issues as well.

One more thing about Mr. Johnson: he came to all our pre-teen parties and blended in with just the right amount of fun and aloofness.

Eighth grade found me back with a female teacher and once again minus my typewriter. It was also the year my father got a new position with his company and the family moved to England for two years. I was torn. Part of me couldn't wait to live amongst the English—from what I saw of them in movies and on TV, they seemed like decent people. But a bigger part of me wanted to stay at Brookville school and graduate with my class.

What to do?

It was during this year, too, that I got my first real taste of a presidential election. It started really in seventh grade with Mr. Johnson, who thought it would be worthwhile for us to know all we could about the election process. After all, one day we, too, would be members of the voting public. Soon the whole class talked of nothing else but the keynote speakers and the party platforms and the nominating speeches. I watched the conventions and knew it was going to be a close race. With the elections on my mind, I couldn't really focus on us moving to London.

And there was the upper-class trip to Washington, D.C. in the spring. I would miss it if I left the states.

I thought again about moving with the family, and about those old Sherlock Holmes movies with Basil Rathbone with their foggy street scenes. My seven-year-old brother was excited, too, but he said he was afraid he wouldn't be able to understand their funny way of speaking. My father assured him that if he could understand the Sherlock Holmes movies, he wouldn't have any trouble understanding the rest of the English population.

It all seemed too good to be true. The prospect of seeing how people in other countries lived, and having a chance to travel abroad—what could be better? People said I couldn't manage life in a foreign country. In my heart, I wanted to go with the family, but I also wanted to finish eighth grade. But after a while, I really had second thoughts. I was in the eighth grade, and in my school, there was a graduation ceremony before starting high school the next year. I had started in the Brookville school system nine years ago as a kindergartner not yet able to walk. And now, here I was in the eighth grade, walking among the many friends I had made. The idea of not being able to see this phase of my life through to its completion, of not being able to graduate with my class, was very upsetting. Besides, I had heard that there was an excellent possibility I would receive the annual good citizenship award that was awarded each year.

With all of this in mind, I persuaded my parents to let me stay behind, living with the Robinsons who were good friends of the family. Although they had five other children, they accepted me into their midst, assuring my parents I wouldn't be a burden. My parents rented their house to a childless couple who were willing to keep our twelve-year-old Newfoundland dog, Muffin. In late December, 1960, with all kinds of mixed emotions, I said good-bye to my mom, my dad and my brother. A new adventure awaited me.

The year before, I had started to wear night braces on both my legs. As I mentioned earlier, when I was a toddler I had night shoes connected to a bar that kept my feet apart—something that was pretty uncomfortable. Now I was wearing two braces, a little more comfortable, but I wasn't able to put them on or take them off by myself. My parents had always done that for me. I was worried about how I would manage without their help. It turned out not to be a problem as putting on the braces became the nightly ritual that was eagerly shared by the three older Robinson children, who also helped by cutting my meat at dinner.

There were, of course, a few minor problems. What bothered me most was that I missed my dog, Muffin. But after some negotiating, an arrangement was made for me to see Muffin at least twice a month and also to see my house and my room with all its familiar objects.

During my six months with the Robinsons, I became an integral part of their family, and I enjoyed my first experience with a Passover Seder.

My parents and my grandparents thought I should go to England as soon as school was over in June. But when the camp application arrived, I insisted that I wanted to go back to Homestead, the sleep-away camp I had loved so much the summer before. This time I wanted to go for the whole summer. Homestead was run by the Unitarian Church. What was lacking in accommodations they more than made up with spirit and heart. I just loved it and made a lifelong friend out of Paul Singer. I'm sure it helped me become the independent person I am today. My reunion with my family would have wait till the end of August.

Soon it was June and graduation day. No one knew who was going to get the good citizenship award, but when the principal said that she wished the parents of the boy who was about to receive the award could be present, I knew that she was talking about me. I had no lack of egotism, and as soon as I heard her words, I started to rise from my seat, all ready to receive the award along with my eighth-grade diploma. Although my parents couldn't be there that day, my grandparents came, and it was such a thrilling moment for me that I knew I had made the right decision to finish the year at my school.

After the ceremony, we all went back to the Robinsons for refreshments and I called my parents to tell them about my award. It was very early morning in London, but I knew my parents would be awake and eager to hear my news firsthand. I thanked them again for letting me stay on and told them I was looking forward to seeing them in August.

Mr. Johnson was at the party and knowing how much I admired Mr. Lincoln, gave me a framed newspaper article with the title, "How Lincoln Did His Best." I still have it hanging in my bedroom today.

A short time later I returned to camp, and again shared a cabin with Paul Singer and spent the night with him and his family during the break between the two sessions.

Looking back on my little adventure away from my family, I see how beneficial it turned out to be. For it prepared me for a life alone.

# London
## August, 1961–June, 1962

I arrived in London at around nine o'clock in the evening. The whole family was there to meet me and welcome me to my new home. My parents knew people who worked for Pan American airlines and they were able to find out who would be piloting my plane to London, since I was traveling by myself at twelve years of age. Overseas planes had very few passengers in those days, the early 60s, so the pilot was free to leave his cabin and spend time with me. I managed to stay awake during the ride into London from the airport, taking in my new environment and wondering if I had made the right choice about staying behind. London looked so magical. Every movie or TV show I had seen regarding the city came alive. I knew I was going to love these next ten months.

No. 29 Palace Gate had three steps leading up to the main entrance. We lived on the sixth floor. Americans would call it the seventh floor, but the English count the first floor as the ground floor. There was a fireplace in the lobby, which I found out later was great on a cold winter morning. The building, which was ninety years old, had the first lift (elevator) ever installed in London. It had outside and inside gates, both of which had to be shut tight before the lift would move. Although I knew the lift wasn't put in with me in mind, it felt as though someone really cared about people with handicaps.

Michael, our chauffeur and general all-around helper, welcomed me to my new home. "I'm glad to meet you, Albert. Your parents have told me so much about you."

"Thank you," I replied. "I'm glad to be here, and I can't wait to see everything."

With that, I was taken on a tour of the apartment. The first rooms I saw were the dining room and the living room. Down a long hall were the bedrooms, and after that was the kitchen, the last room in this huge apartment. This meant that when food was served, it had to be rushed through the apartment on a trolley to get to the dining room before it got cold. And cold the apartment often was. There was no central heating in the whole building. We had to rely totally on electric heaters in each room, but electricity was so expensive that most of the time they were turned off and we learned to wear sweaters. My mother's knitting sure came in handy.

Soon I had to use the bathroom, which again was at the end of the long hall, not that convenient for someone like me who had trouble walking. When I got there, I sat down on the seat, only to give out a little shout, for the seat was so cold. I don't imagine that many people sat there reading the newspaper.

From there, I had to go to an adjoining room to wash my hands. The only good thing about the whole experience was the heated towel rack. I guess there should be some compensation when you have to put up with all that cold.

When I finally joined the family again outside my bedroom, my mother said, "We heard your scream of surprise. Now you can join us in our little game. You see, we all keep quiet when guests go to enter the loo." When I looked puzzled, she said, "That's what the English call their small toilet."

"Very funny," I said.

"And what do you think of the washbasin and bathtub being in a separate room?"

"I kinda like it," I replied. "I guess the English figured it's nice to be able to wash their hands without having to deal with their smell."

"And do you know, Albert," my brother exclaimed, "I even have a sink in my room."

"With a heated towel rack?" I exclaimed.

"Of course," he replied. "We English have to have some warmth before we put our faces out into the cold world. Of course, you're still an American, so you don't have a sink in your room."

"Well, at least I got the bigger room."

We all laughed. Sibling rivalry hadn't died, despite our eight-month separation.

"It's getting late," my mother exclaimed. "I'd love to stay up all night and talk to you, but you must be exhausted from your trip."

"I'm afraid I am, so I'll see you all in the morning," I replied as I entered my room.

The room was indeed huge, and I loved the big picture window. I was only sorry that it was up too high for me to sit on the window sill and look out at the view below of the street, Palace Gate. I soon became fascinated by the glow of the streetlights, and the funny sounds of the diesel engines of the London taxis. This was my first experience living in a city, as before that day I had spent my entire life in the country, with all its stillness and dark nights.

I unpacked my suitcase and took out the engraved traveling clock that had been my prize at graduation. On the top it said, "Award for Good Citizenship, June, 1961."

I thought back to the wonderful time I had just had, sharing the lives of another family for six months, even though I'd had to share a very small room with the two boys in the family. How I wished all the Robinsons could see me now, in my huge English room and still-strange apartment. I could see it was going to be a year full of all kinds of new experiences.

The next morning I got up early and had breakfast with my father. He no longer had to rush to take the commuter train, but now that we lived and worked in London, he drove to his office, with Michael sitting beside him. Michael then drove the car back to the apartment, ready to take my mother and my brother and me wherever we wanted to go. Even though my mother had managed to drive quite successfully back home, despite her polio, she decided that negotiating unfamiliar London streets, with cars driving on the left, would be too much for her. My dad had no problems, though, and on weekends he drove the family all around the surrounding countryside.

When Michael returned that morning, my mother decided to take me on a tour of the neighborhood and to her favorite store, Harrods. As I started to get into the car, opening the door on the right, my mother and Michael both yelled, "Other side! Other side!"

"Oh, yes," I said. "I forgot."

"Well, you'd better remember," my mother exclaimed. "Even crossing the street, you must always look right. Last week a foreign diplomat forgot and looked left. He was hit by a car and killed."

"Yikes! I'd better remember that," I replied, thinking that my time in London was truly going to be quite an adventure.

As we drove along and I looked out the window at all the ancient buildings, I thought how lucky I was to be driving through centuries of history. I knew that each little mews we passed had a different story to tell. My mother pointed out the Albert Memorial. "I'm sorry to have to tell you it's not named after you."

"It's not? You mean you didn't tell them I was coming?"

"No, I'm afraid Queen Victoria had already decided to name the memorial after her husband, Prince Albert. And look, across the street is the Royal Albert Hall. It's a great concert hall. In fact, we're going there next week. I was able to get tickets for the Pete Seeger concert."

"That's great," I replied excitedly. "I really like him—and the Weavers, too. We sang a lot of their songs at camp."

I continued to enjoy the view of all the low rise buildings, most of which were no more than four stories high. I found out later that there was a building code that didn't allow buildings in that area to be built above a certain height in order to prevent occupants from looking into Buckingham Palace.

Our one and only stop that day was Harrods, the famous department store. Harrods was situated across from a square with a quaint mews, which is what the British call their charming little alleys. It had a few stylish boutiques and several restaurants. They would have to wait for another day to be explored. Today we were going to Harrods.

When we arrived, Michael got out the wheelchair from the "boot" of the car and my mother got into it. This would be my maiden voyage of pushing my mother around in her wheelchair. She seemed unconcerned, but I was a bit nervous.

"Please come back for us at four," my mother exclaimed to Michael.

Four? I looked at my watch and saw that it was only ten. What in the world would we be doing in a store for six hours?

Entering the store, my mother said, "Look at the directory over here. You'll see you can buy everything here—from a sewing needle to a rack of venison. You can even rent a farm in Wales from their estate office here. In fact, this is where Dad and I found our flat. Now, what part of the store would you like to see first?"

My mind was racing back and forth between food and books and the art gallery and clothes and buying theater tickets. I chose food. Not a restaurant, we'd do that later, but the Food Hall. There we saw an incredible assortment of beautifully arranged fruits and vegetables and poultry (including quail and pigeons and goose) and meats (including rabbit and antelope). The meat was cut by butchers dressed in white ties and tails. It was all incredible. I felt like I was in an art gallery waiting for Picasso to appear at any moment.

Our plan was to start on the ground floor with the Food Hall and then work our way upward, ending up on the fourth floor, the top, where we'd have lunch and go to the art gallery and the theater booking office.

"Sounds good to me," I said, still amazed at all the things one could purchase in one place. The only thing missing was a hotel where we could find a room to take a nap when we became exhausted, as I was sure we would.

Using the elevators to go up to each floor, I was pleased at how well we managed together. In those days, I could walk for miles. Today, so many years later, it's very hard for me to walk even a full city block.

When we got to the meat department, my mother was greeted by the head butcher. "Nigel," she exclaimed, "I want you to meet my son, Albert. He just arrived from America last night."

"It's an honor to meet you, young man," Nigel replied.

"Nigel is the person who makes sure we get our bacon and meat cut the way we like it," my mother explained.

"I do my best, madam," Nigel replied. "I know you like the rind off the bacon and the bone removed. I know just how you like your Sunday roasts."

"Nigel is also responsible for getting the royal family their meat. That's why he is all dressed up in his white tie and tails."

"Well, you're a queen, mother, too," I exclaimed.

"Well, at least I am at Palace Gate," she answered.

Leaving the Food Hall, we began to explore all the other wonderful sections of the store. I especially loved the book department, which contained both new and secondhand books. Here I learned that books that were more than six months old were marked down as secondhand books, something that made it easy for me to buy lots of books there during my year in England. I also found that if I wanted a book that they didn't stock, they would advertise for it and usually get it for me.

I was getting the hang of pushing Mother in her chair, which turned out to be good for me, too, as it gave me something to hang on to. During the many times I pushed her in her wheelchair that year, I never lost my balance and rarely felt tired after one of our long walks.

Soon it was time for lunch, and Mother dragged me away from the books and we went to one of the top floor restaurants. Although my mother tried to interest me in all kinds of typically English food, I opted for the English version of a hamburger, which was served in a hard roll and tasted very un-American, though quite edible.

The day ended with a visit to Harrods theater ticket booking office where my mother purchased four orchestra tickets (the English call them "stall" seats) for a new musical, *Oliver*. This was the first and only time the whole family would attend a theatrical performance together.

Taking the elevator down to the ground floor, I glanced at my watch. It was 3:45 and almost time to meet Michael.

"You sure fooled me," I exclaimed to my mother. "I can't believe we've been here all this time."

"I know, and there are still things we haven't seen. We'll have to come back again and see the art gallery."

We arrived home at the same time as my father, who every day took advantage of the long English summer days which stayed light until almost ten. He would walk home from his office through the Kensington Gardens, a large and beautiful park near our home.

At dinner that night, I got my first taste of what life is like when one has a kitchen in one part of the house and the dining room in the other. It was a comical sight, for there was Michael, all dressed up in a shirt, tie and white jacket, racing down two long corridors with our dinner resting on a not-too-sturdy-looking glass tea trolley. But despite my apprehensions, Michael and the food arrived intact. However, the layout of the apartment would remain a puzzle in my mind.

After dinner, we all retired to the den, which was next to the kitchen, and where we would eat our meals on Michael's days off. There we would watch the rented "telly," the TV. The free BBC channel we all enjoyed was not really free, as everyone in England had to purchase a TV license to pay for the channel.

In those days, the English had only two TV channels—the BBC and one commercial channel. I especially like the American programs, like *Perry Mason*, which were uninterrupted by commercials. It was fun to watch the BBC logo of a black and white globe which spun around after each program.

The days flew by, and soon it was Thursday, the day my mother and I were to attend the Pete Seeger concert at Royal Albert Hall. It would also be my first test of pushing my mother in her wheelchair on the crowded London sidewalks. By this time, I was feeling pretty confident that I could manage.

"Can you believe you've been here a week already?" my mother said as we slowly made our way down Palace Gate.

"No," I said, "I can't. In fact, it seems much longer. I'm starting to feel right at home here—in spite of all the stairs we both have to negotiate just to get into our building."

"I know, but we really do manage quite well with all the help we get."

Continuing down the street, we came to the first curb. It was high and I knew I wouldn't be able to maneuver the wheelchair down and then back up. My mother was not at all concerned. She simply got out of the wheelchair and, tipping it back, got it down into the street. Then she got herself back into the chair and I pushed her across the street until we reached the sidewalk curb, where once again my mother surprised the curious onlookers by getting out of the chair again.

"Pretty nifty, isn't it?" my mother said to anyone in earshot.

Reaching Albert Hall, we left the wheelchair in the lobby, and a nice couple helped us up the stairs, and then the ushers helped us to our seats in the huge auditorium.

"Turn around, Albert," my mother said. "Look at the gold crown above the box behind us. That's where the queen sits when she attends a concert."

A chill came over me as I thought about all the history I was witnessing almost everywhere I went in London. When I had been in Washington, D.C. with my class, I had also felt a part of history when I saw the memorials to Washington,

Jefferson and Lincoln. But most of America, with its relative newness, and its pioneering tradition of forever changing and always growing, never gave me this same sense I had in London of witnessing the important landmarks and the symbols of hundreds of years of history.

But soon Pete Seeger appeared and I found myself carried away with emotion for America when he sang "This Land Is Your Land" and "We Shall Overcome."

The concert was wonderful and at the end, the audience stood while we sang "The Star-Spangled Banner" and "God Save the Queen." The ushers helped us down the steps and to the wheelchair. As we made our way back to the apartment, I was struck by all the kindness we were shown by people who, when seeing my mother getting out of her chair at each curb, would insist on helping so she could remain seated.

The next real adventure started that Saturday when the whole family left for a three-week tour of the European continent. I was so excited about the prospect of seeing the places I'd read about in books or seen depicted in movies. Of course, all that would have to wait until the plane landed. And this was no ordinary plane—or it wouldn't be considered ordinary now. Believe it or not, our car actually went on the plane, too. It was put in the baggage section, along with three other cars and everyone's luggage. (I guess it was a specially built plane, and that renting cars abroad was not such an easy thing to do in 1961.)

Our first stop was Amsterdam, where we checked into our hotel and then took a sightseeing boat that toured the canals. I have always been attracted to water, in all forms, but it wasn't until three years later, and another continent away, that I realized this. But that day in Amsterdam, I was content to just ride along, listening to our guide telling us about the rich history of the city.

I remembered reading *The Diary of a Young Girl* in junior high school, and now our canal boat took us directly past the building where Anne Frank and her family had lived until the Nazis found them and took them away.

As we drove along, we found a delicatessen for lunch. It was the start of three weeks of picnicking in the car. Sitting in the back, I was all set to enjoy the feast, which was easy for me, as the car we had rented came equipped with two dropleaf tables.

Of course, there were times when we didn't get what we thought we had ordered. In Germany we saw a sign saying "Hambergers sold here." Well, you would have thought that the family had struck gold, the way all four of our faces lit up with excitement. Mouths watering, we waited for our "hamburgers." Alas, what we were served were not hamburgers but omelettes cooked with strips of ham. My father took the man behind the counter to the sign in the shop window and pointed to the word "hamberger."

"Yes," the man replied with a smile, pointing to our omelettes. "Hamberger."

This, of course, was in the pre-McDonald days. So, disappointed, we thanked him and, retreating to the car, we decided to eat the omelettes in the car anyway. Luckily, they were delicious.

But back to Holland. The remainder of our first day there was spent napping and shopping. The day ended with my dictating my diary to my brother. This was the first of a daily activity. I couldn't write clearly without a typewriter, so my brother quite willingly wrote down for me a record of what we did and, also, of my thoughts.

The next day we were off on a real adventure.

Back in London, before our trip to Holland, Michael would often take my mother on various excursions throughout the city. One day he took her to the National Gallery of Art and it was there that she fell in love with paintings of the modern Dutch painter, Everson, who, although still alive at the time, painted in the style of the old Dutch Masters. After getting Mr. Everson's address in Holland, my mother wrote to him, saying that she and her family would be in Holland and she would be honored if she could meet him.

Mr. Everson wrote back, inviting us to his house and sending us directions. So, on our second day in Holland, right after our continental breakfast of orange juice, milk and croissants, we were off.

Despite Mr. Everson's directions, we still managed to get lost. To this day, I can hear my father asking the way and being told "straight on." Over the years, this phrase has remained in our family vocabulary and the words "straight on" are uttered whenever any of us is asked for directions. (Funny what can happen when you don't speak the language and are without a phrase book.) Anyway, we finally found the house and, it seems, none too soon, for as we drove into the driveway, whom did we find but Mr. Everson, with golf clubs in his hand, walking out his front door. Another example of miscommunication, perhaps due to the language barrier, as he forgot the time for our visit, or did not understand in the first place. Luckily my father was able to persuade him to delay his game and show us his studio.

I remember walking into a room with an easel on which was a painting of a plate with fruit. The fruit looked so real that I wanted to take a bite out of one of the apples. What made the experience even more fascinating was to see how Mr. Everson painted his subjects, for hanging from the ceiling, suspended by heavy string, were various pieces of fruit. The resulting mobile was a picture in itself.

The whole family fell in love with the painting, and it wasn't long before Mr. Everson accepted my father's offer to buy it and took out his paintbrush to add some final touches to his work.

Before we left, Mr. Everson told us that we had bought one of six paintings he would create that year. My parents invited him to visit us in London so that he could see his work displayed. He thanked us and told us he planned to be in London early in the new year.

With that, we were off to Germany, and Mr. Everson was off to his game of golf, a little more money now in his hand.

Our next major stop was Düsseldorf, but not before some fancy driving by my father over the Swiss Alps. Sometimes we were driving behind huge trucks carrying cars, their rear ends swaying back and forth over the narrow roads that clung to the sides of the Alps. It was amazing to me that the trucks never went over the edge, and that our car, too, stayed upright. To me, it was even more remarkable since we were driving an English car, designed for the "wrong" side of the road.

We reached Düsseldorf on a Saturday afternoon, too late for my mother to do any shopping. My father was, of course, delighted, and this too became a family joke. From that time on, he always tried to time our visits to major cities and their shopping centers when the shops were already closed.

The next day we set off early on the Autobahn, the German superhighway. The Autobahn had no speed limits, so my father was zipping speedily along, hoping we would reach our destination in the Black Forest by lunchtime. To his surprise, in a short time he spotted a sign announcing the end of the Autobahn. We had driven too far—in fact, ninety miles too far. So my father simply turned around and headed back. One of the good things about a highway that has no speed restrictions is that ninety miles can be made up in no time at all.

Finally we were at our hotel, which was situated on a lake in the wooded mountain region of southwest Germany, one of the most beautiful spots I have ever seen. We would spend five days there, just swimming and having fun by the water, and, it turned out, the one and only time that I would ever spend a large chunk of time at a seaside resort.

My swimming was really coming along. My father, surprised to see how well I was doing and how far I could swim, paid me one of his rare compliments. "Albert," he exclaimed, "I'm amazed. I didn't know you had become such a good swimmer."

Every afternoon, along with the swimming, came motor boating around the lake. In my mind, that ranked right alongside swimming as one of my favorite things to do. Meanwhile, my brother was having a wonderful time playing with all kinds of kids. The fact that no one spoke the same language didn't really seem to matter. Just having fun was the important rule of the day.

The hotel reminded me of a hunting lodge, similar to the ones you might find scattered around New England. It became the stage for a memorable tenth birthday party for my brother.

The day before his birthday, my parents approached the hotel's maitre d', telling him that it would be their son's birthday the next day and that they would like a special Black Forest cake made up for four people to mark the occasion.

Well, the big day arrived, and out came a beautiful Black Forest cake, all done up with birthday candles. The only trouble was its size. Instead of being a cake for four people, as my parents had instructed, it was a huge cake, big enough to feed the entire hotel. And that, in fact, is exactly what we did. My brother took a piece of cake over to everyone he had played with on the beach. It didn't take long for one of the German girls to realize what was happening, for she quickly excused herself and returned in a few minutes with a little stuffed animal for my brother.

The next morning we said good-bye to the Black Forest and headed once again in the direction of the Swiss Alps. Our goal, which we achieved, was to have our lunch overlooking Lake Geneva. Like all of our drives through Switzerland, this one was truly breathtaking in its beauty, and I made a pact with myself to return to Switzerland when I was older. I did manage to return twice to Lucerne, but alas, no more.

After lunch we went on a tour through the League of Nations. Before we started out on our trip, I had written to the League. I explained my interest in current events, told them when we would be in Geneva, and asked if it would be possible to take a guided tour. With the confirming letter in hand, we spent part of the afternoon touring the League of Nations. I was in heaven, as it made my current history lessons come alive.

The next morning, with some sadness and excitement, we said our farewell to Switzerland, and making our way again across the Alps, we said hello to Venice, Italy.

It was quite an experience for me to see a whole city surrounded by water. The city was both beautiful and dirty at the same time. All kinds of debris floated in the water, including a dead rat. Still, it was fun riding in a water taxi to the hotel, and entering the front lobby not from the front street but from a boat dock. And of course we had to ride around like typical tourists in a gondola, and had our pictures taken, too.

The best shots of all were taken by my father in St. Mark's Square. There we are—my mother and I. She is in a wheelchair and I am standing behind her, pushing it, and both of us are surrounded by pigeons eating crusts of bread at our feet. An even better picture was taken of my brother with pigeons clinging to various parts of his body.

At the same time we were enjoying our bird friends, we had to keep watch over our wallets, as the larger two-legged animals were out to get us everywhere. If they didn't literally pick your pockets, they did figuratively with their sky-high prices. We were shocked to see what a glass of Coke went for in the square. And if that wasn't bad enough, there were several times that we were shortchanged.

Luckily, we did manage to enjoy dinner on the Hotel Danieli roof garden. Along with delicious food, we were treated to a spectacular view of the canals at night.

The next morning, even though we were still in Venice, we went by car on dry land to the Lido, as the beach was called. Here we swam in clear, unpolluted water. It was wonderful. As you can gather, I didn't really care much for Venice and was glad when we left the next morning for Florence.

Again we were driving on the "wrong" side of the road for our English car, but all went well. We had a picnic lunch of cheese and crackers, for this time we were not fooled by any signs, and we picked out the food ourselves.

We arrived in Florence in the early afternoon and were shown to our rooms. At this particular hotel, we not only had two adjacent rooms, but two balconies as well. The view would have been wonderful, but Florence was in the middle of a very serious drought, and the Arno River, which ran alongside our hotel, was completely dry. Still, we all enjoyed having our continental breakfast seated on the balcony.

I fell in love with Florence and knew that I had to return to this marvelous city some day, for a visit of two days could never be enough to see everything I wanted to see.

The city was steeped in the culture of the Renaissance of the fourteenth to sixteenth centuries. There was a replica of Michelangelo's David in one of the squares, and when my father took a picture of my mother and me standing next to it, my mother said, "If you think this is great, wait till we get to Rome and we have another picture taken next to the original."

Before we left Florence, the whole family went shopping. First we visited the famous Florentine leather factories where I bought my first brown leather wallet. It made me feel like a real grown-up. And for some reason, I found myself telling the salesman how much I loved his city and about the dry river next to our hotel.

"Yes, isn't that something," he said, smiling. "And in Italian, a river is called *fiumi*."

"A dry *fiumi*," my father said, and we all laughed, including the salesman. There was something about the sound of those two words that we found amusing. Maybe it was because it sounded like a "dry martini"—or maybe there was another reason, but from that moment, the Elias family had a new phrase that we added to "Straight on!"

The next things we bought were hats, great big yellow ones with long beaks on which college students stuck whatever awards they had won during their university days. I wished that I, too, was in college, but I was going to have to wait four more years before I could have some awards of my own.

My mother was in heaven at our next stop, for it was here that my father bought her a necklace with a beautiful diamond in the center. The necklace needed to have some adjustments made and would be delivered to us at our hotel, the Excelsior.

After a wonderful day of exploring the city, we were having dinner in the hotel dining room when a messenger walked in with a small package for my mother. It was her necklace, and she put on the necklace right then and there. It was gorgeous and fit perfectly. Everyone *oohed* and *ahhed*. Everyone, that is, except my ten-year-old brother. "Mommie," he exclaimed in a loud voice, "why is there only one diamond in front? Daddy should have bought you a necklace with diamonds going all the way around." Everyone laughed, but that didn't interfere with my mother's radiant smile.

The next morning we said our good-byes to Florence, but both my brother and I swore to return there one day. My brother even wrote to the Excelsior Hotel in 1983, hoping they would remember him and the number of the room we had been in back in 1960. But alas, the hotel's records didn't go back that far. They were happy that he remembered them and offered him another room. Somehow, he never returned to Florence, but I made it back twice, once in the summer of 1965 when my parents gave me a trip to Europe as a graduation present and again in 2001 with my friend Susan. I can still remember sitting on the grass during an outdoor concert at the Pitti Palace, home of the Medici family during the Renaissance and now an art museum.

Leaving Florence, we were on our way to Rome. My father told us that he would splurge and hire a guide for the full three days we were there as there was just so much to see.

I thought that was great, but at the same time I couldn't stop thinking about the Eversen painting we had just bought. I told my father I wanted to hang it up in each of the remaining hotel rooms. But my father said no. "You'll have a life-time to admire Mr. Eversen's fruit. Wait another week or so, until we're back in England, and you'll see it then. In the meantime, just be content holding the treasure in the backseat."

"We feel the same way, dear," my mother replied. "But now that we'll be in the car for a few hours, why don't you boys tell your Daddy and me what you've liked best about the trip so far."

I spoke first, telling them how fascinated I was with our visit with Mr. Eversen, and about his telling me that because he used real fruit, he had to work really fast so that he could complete his painting before they spoiled.

"You really had quite a conversation with him," my mother exclaimed. "But one thing he forgot to tell you, but he mentioned to me, was that he had studied the details of how the old Dutch masters mixed their paints so that his work really looked like theirs."

"I'm glad you appreciate art, Albert," my father replied. "If you're good, per-haps Mother will take you to the Royal Academy when we get back to London. There you can see the work of lots of the Dutch masters."

"That would be wonderful," I exclaimed.

"Good," Mother answered. "Now let's hear from the birthday boy. What was the highlight of our trip for you so far?"

"Playing on the beach, my birthday party, and having the family's picture taken with the Polar Bear."

"The picture with the Polar Bear?" I exclaimed. "I would never have picked that as a highlight of anything.

"Now Albert," Mother replied, "that's not nice. Everyone is entitled to their own opinion. And your brother will remember celebrating his birthday in Titisee for many years to come."

"Titisee?" I asked. I thought we were in the Black Forest."

"We were," Father replied, "but Titisee was the town in the Black Forest."

"Oh," I exclaimed, "thanks for telling me. I guess I'll always remember Titisee, too, but for the lake and the fun we had in the boats."

"Yes," Mother replied. "And I'll always remember the hotel we stayed at with the grass growing on its lower roof. It reminded me of a Swiss chateau."

"A Swiss chateau?" I replied. "It reminded me of a New England hunting lodge."

"That's okay, too," Mother answered. "It doesn't matter as long as you remember the trip. That's what counts."

All eyes were on my father now. It was his turn to speak. What would he say? What were his fondest memories of the trip?

Just as he was about to speak, however, we saw a sign saying "Welcome to Rome." Would we get lost here, too? Father was taking no chances, and stopped the car on the side of the road. As he got out of the car, a bread truck pulled up and my father asked the driver the way to the Hotel Hassler. Unfortunately, the driver didn't speak English and my father didn't speak Italian. Nevertheless, my father proceeded to repeat every word the driver said, not understanding any of them. We were all hysterical with laughter and decided the best thing to do was to just go "straight on." We were bound to find the hotel sooner or later. But because of this, we never did find out what Father considered the highlight of the trip. But I think that besides the purchase of the Eversen painting, it was the appreciation of different languages and their often funny-sounding words that we encountered.

It was around four in the afternoon when we finally reached our hotel. This time we had rooms on two different floors. Before we went our separate ways, it was decided to meet in our parents' room for cocktails at 6:30. Entering our rooms, however, our plans quickly changed. Normally, it was our parents who got the hotel's suite, but not this time.

In those days, back in 1960, hotels had keys—not the plastic computerized cards—and the Hotel Hassler had their keys mounted on a red wooden slab with the name of the hotel written on it in gold lettering. (It was so beautiful that I couldn't help myself and kept my key as a treasured souvenir.) So that day, when my brother and I used our key to open our door, we discovered, much to our delight, that we were given the suite and our parents were given the small "chauffeur's room." They were really good sports about it and didn't demand a swap. However, we did allow them to enter our room each night, providing they brought the drinks. But it was the birthday boy who called room service and ordered the ice.

One of the great features of our room was its huge bathtub, and my brother took full advantage of it. Every night before he took his bath he would get on top of the bathroom sink and then dive into the tub. Even though it looked dangerous, and he could have been seriously hurt, I envied his ability to do this. I had to be content to just lie in the "small pool" and kick my legs and move my arms, without doing the laps I would have done in a real pool.

(William was indeed lucky in Rome, but it hadn't always been that way. I can remember several occasions back home in the States when I had to call to get an ambulance to rush him to the nearest hospital emergency room because he had dressed up as Superman and jumped off one of our end tables only to hit some part of his face or head against the coffee table. I understand that two of his sons are doing the same thing today. Now he knows what he put me through so many years ago.)

But back to Rome. The guide my parents hired was wonderful, and again, with my father doing the driving, it was always "straight on!"

I think my favorite memory of Rome's tourist attractions was Michelangelo's statue of Moses. Legend has it that when Michelangelo finished carving Moses, he was so full of emotion that he looked into the marble eyes of the creation and said, "Moses, speak to me!" When nothing came from the statue's lips, he got so mad that he hit his masterpiece's knee with his chisel. After my mother told me this story, I made it a point to look long at Moses's face. My father bought my brother and me miniature statues of both David and Moses, but alas, some forty years later, only David has survived my many moves.

My mother still loves "her David," and insisted that my father take a picture of her with me and my brother. This is my mother's favorite shot.

Another sight I will long remember is the Forum. I could just picture the ancient Romans doing battle in the square. However, there were hundreds of wild cats living in the Forum and my mother could hardly wait to get away from there because of her fear of cats.

At the end of each day, we said good-bye to our professional guide and left the remainder of that day's tour to the amateur, namely, my father. I must say that this time he did good and got us to Harry's Bar at the bottom of the Spanish Steps. At last the family could enjoy a good old American hamburger. There were other Americans at the restaurant so we were able to catch up on all the latest news and gossip from back in the U.S.A. An expatriate had a good idea when he opened the bar, because no matter how much you enjoy visiting or living in another country, there are times when you long for the things that remind you of home. (Something that would ring true to me during the next year in London.)

After that night's triumph, we were all on the edge of our car seats to see how my father would top Harry's Bar the following night. We had decided to go "native" and have a real Italian meal. What gave the night an even greater flavor of adventure was the decision to leave the car behind and go by taxi.

So, there we all were, the four of us seated in the backseat of the cab, not speaking a word of Italian, but somehow conveying to our driver our desire for some real Italian food. The driver drove (always "straight on!") for about forty-five minutes, and stopped the cab in front of an outdoor restaurant called Alfredo's. We had all heard of the famous Alfredo chain of restaurants all over

Rome. But this one was quite different and was not on the tourist map. The outdoor tables were surrounded by tenement buildings, all with balconies. We never did find out the name of the town we were in, but it was surely on the outskirts of Rome. Perhaps our driver lived there. One thing was sure, we were all extremely hungry.

We were shown to a table which was located right in the middle of the square.

"Well, boys," my father exclaimed, "this is not the Alfredo's your mother and I wanted to take you to."

"It's not?" I asked.

"No," Mother replied, backing up my father.

"But Mom," I exclaimed, "it's so Italian. Just listen to those two women shouting at each other from the balconies."

We laughed as all heads looked up at the women. The women's hands as well as their mouths were going a mile a minute.

"Oh, well," Father replied, "as long as the food tastes as good as the Alfredo's in Rome, I'm willing to put up with two women expressing themselves." He paused and looked at us before continuing. "But only for one night."

We assured him that for our last night in Rome we would find a restaurant close to the hotel, if not in it.

Soon the waiter brought out our dinners. It would be the first time I tasted fettuccine alfredo. I really enjoyed it and from then on would order it whenever I was dining in an Italian restaurant. (Oh, if only I had known that the rich cream sauce contributed to my gallbladder trouble, I might have switched to Italian veal or mushroom dishes much earlier.) Since I only have the use of my left hand and as a result holding both a knife and a fork at the same time is impossible, the waiter cut up the noodles for me, a job usually reserved for my father.

Everyone enjoyed their meal, but when it came time to leave, my father got up from the table and a nail from the leg of the chair tore a hole in his trousers, putting a damper on what had been a very delightful dinner.

Two days later we said our good-byes to Rome and headed in the direction of the Italian Riviera. We all needed a rest on the beach after the hectic few days in Rome.

Up to this point, my father had made all the hotel reservations, but this particular spot he had left in the hands of a British travel agent. Boy, he wished he hadn't. When we arrived at the hotel, the whole family looked at one another, wondering what we were getting ourselves into.

My father instructed my mother and me to stay in the car while he and my brother went inside the hotel to investigate. They soon returned and exclaimed, "We're not staying here as both the dining room and public toilets are filthy."

"Oh, my," Mother replied. "Where can we stay then, dear?"

My father looked at all of us and said, "I thought we'd show the boys Pisa and Portofino."

"Now you boys can say you saw the leaning tower of Pisa."

"Oh!" I said excitedly. "I've heard you and Daddy talk so much about the tower and Portofino. It will be fun for William and me to finally see them for ourselves."

We drove on for a few more hours. I was enjoying the Italian countryside with its olive trees and hills when my father pulled the car into a town square. "Look boys," he said. "Look straight ahead of you. What do you see?"

William and I both looked in the direction he was pointing.

"Look, Albert," William exclaimed excitedly. "Look at the tower. It's really leaning. I wish we could climb it."

We both looked at our parents, hoping this could happen.

"William," Father said, "you and I will walk up the stairs to the top. Albert and Mother will take the elevator to the first landing and wait for us to come down."

Though disappointed that I wasn't included in the expedition to the top of the tower, I did manage to have an enjoyable view of the city and to keep Mother company. The elevator didn't travel to the top, and neither of us was any good when it came to climbing stairs. But our day in the sun was soon to come.

Just before we left the tower, my mother and I leaned against the fence that surrounded it. In fact, I was leaning against my mother so it looked like we were perfectly "straight" and the leaning tower and everyone else was off center. My father thought that it was funny and snapped our picture. It was one of the most memorable ones from the trip. The best shot, however, was awaiting us in Portofino.

A few hours later, we said good-bye to Pisa and continued our journey down the Italian coast, arriving in Portofino around dinnertime. We immediately made our way to the Splendido Hotel, which was situated at the top of a hill and had a spectacular view of the Mediterranean. We all got a kick out of the buses as they went down the hill, their funny horns a-blazing to other vehicles as they navigated the curves on the narrow road.

Portofino was a true vacation because for two days nobody knew where we were. And the four of us were not in the mood to announce to our family and friends the last-minute change in hotel reservations. So we were free to lose ourselves amongst the fishermen of the Mediterranean.

I loved the fishing boats and was given free run of the pier. I had my favorite picture taken seated on cement steps looking out at the vast expanse of water and wishing that I could be on a boat, too. But it was not to be, at least not on this trip. I would have to wait four more years before I would take an extended sea voyage.

The personnel at the Splendido couldn't have been nicer. The waiters in the dining room took great pride in helping me cut my meat and making sure that everything was to my liking.

I was really sad when our two days ended, and I promised myself that I would return one day. But so far, Portofino is just a memory—a strong memory, because I can still hear those buses tooting their amusing horns as they headed down the hill toward the Mediterranean.

Paris was our next stop. Again William and I lucked out with the hotel room. This time, in the Hotel Ares Eiffel, we had a duplex suite overlooking the Eiffel Tower. The duplex had a balcony and I especially enjoyed sitting out at night looking at the Tower and seeing Paris all aglow.

When Mom and Dad saw our excitement with our suite, my father said, "We thought we would stay at a hotel in Paris that is frequented by the English. It's not as expensive as the hotels that cater to Americans. We wanted to teach you boys thrift by staying at a less fancy place. But, looking at the two of you now, I can see we seem to have failed. Oh, well. C'est la vie."

"Don't say you failed," William exclaimed. "Just think how happy you've made Albert. He loves the Hotel Ares Eiffel and he can get up and down the stairs with no trouble. And he loves it out on the balcony. We're going to sit out there tonight and Albert's going to write in his diary."

"Well," Dad replied, "enjoy it while you can. I guess living like kings for two nights can't hurt you. Just remember that life won't always be this plush."

There was silence and our parents left, hoping that we got the message.

The next morning we visited the Louvre and saw the Mona Lisa. If it weren't for all the fuss made over Mona's famous smile, I would probably have walked right by it. Oh well, that's show biz.

In the afternoon, while Mother shopped and then napped, I took William and Dad on a little adventure.

I have always been fascinated by detective stories, loving Sherlock Holmes, and had already visited the FBI headquarters in Washington. Now, since I was in Paris, why not visit Interpol? Before coming to Paris, I had written them, giving the dates of our visit. To everyone's surprise, they wrote back to say that if I brought along their letter, they would be happy to show me around. I gave my father the letter, and after he presented it to them, we were taken on a tour of this international crime-fighting center.

It was mostly room after room of files, but I was still interested in seeing how the agency linked up with police departments all over the world. This was forty-six years ago. Just think what it's like now with e-mail and the Internet.

The next day we were off again, this time to Amiens on the French coast. Our whirlwind tour was at an end, for Amiens was where we would be catching the ferry that would take us across the English Channel and back to 29 Palace Gate.

It had been quite a trip. Every form of transportation had been utilized, except the train. It was the one and only time I would ever see cars and people traveling on the same airplane. And it would be the one and only time the whole family would be away together on any kind of a vacation.

I did manage to travel back to Europe on many occasions. But now, so many years later, with a major loss of mobility, I know that my free and easy European travel days are at an end. Is that the reason I remember every little detail of a trip I took at the age of thirteen?

29 Palace Gate looked good that Saturday night we arrived. Although we had had a wonderful time, it was good to be home. I was especially excited because Monday was the first day of my new school.

I would be a freshman in high school. The very thought of high school made me feel very grown-up. And to be going to a high school in a foreign country made me feel that I was entering a world surrounded with an aura of mystery.

Sunday morning we were back in Kensington Gardens. I pushed Mother's wheelchair over to the pond so that she could feed the ducks. I looked forward to resuming these weekly walks. On our way back to our flat—I was learning to use this English term for our apartment—I spotted a man walking a Newfoundland dog and soon I was thinking about Muffin. Was she being properly looked after? Would she remember me? And with a lump in my throat, I wondered if she'd still be alive when we arrived back home in the States. She was thirteen, an old age for most dogs, but especially for Newfoundland dogs who usually don't live past eight or nine.

That afternoon, I was initiated into an English tradition: Sunday high tea.

At around 3:30, my parents told my brother and me to start putting on our shirts and ties. We would be leaving in forty-five minutes.

"Where are we going?" I asked my brother.

"You'll see," he replied. "Just put on a nice shirt and a jacket."

"No tie?" I asked.

"Of course a tie, stupid."

He had forgotten that I couldn't manage a tie by myself.

When my father came in to see if we were ready and I told him why I wasn't wearing a tie, he said, "I know it's almost impossible to do it with only one hand, so I've come to help you."

In the early 1960s, there were no clip-on ties, so this was the beginning of an almost daily ritual of my father helping me put on a tie, as the American School in London required all the male students to wear ties every day. When I came back to the States, I went to a private school for two years that also required a tie. (In my adult life, I sometimes use clip-on ties, but I also use ties that have been pre-tied, but very loosely, and I put them over my head and tighten them with one hand. I get a better selection of ties that way, and I can manage to loosen them in order to take them off.)

That afternoon in London, I thanked my father for his help and then we were both silent, deep in our own thoughts. Finally my father said, "Don't worry, Albert. Just ask me or your brother if you need help." There was another silence, and then my father said, "Okay?"

"Okay," I said.

After a short car ride, we pulled into a circular driveway and stopped in front of the entrance to the Savoy Hotel.

"What are we doing here?" I asked.

"You'll see," William replied.

"We're introducing you to a typical English Sunday," my mother said. I soon learned that this was really a typical upper class English Sunday, and not that typical, as most English people had their high teas at home.

"Remember," my mother continued, "when I told you that we were going to move to London, I said that the only person I knew there was the doorman at the Savoy? Well, that's why we're starting with the Savoy. But we'll introduce you to a different hotel every Sunday."

We were soon seated at a table in a beautiful dining room and when the waiter came over to take our order, my mother said, "Cecil, I want you to meet our oldest son, Albert."

"A pleasure, Madam," Cecil replied. "But I hope he isn't like his brother and father and orders milk instead of tea."

"I'm afraid he is," Mother replied. "I'm the only adventurous one."

"Then milk it is," answered Cecil. "Now, what kind of sandwiches can I bring you?"

"I'll have cucumber and tomato," Mother replied. "And toast also, thank you."

"Toast?" I asked.

"Yes, toast," my mother replied. "This is going to be our dinner, too. High tea is served as the evening meal."

We all decided to order what my mother had chosen, and then my brother said, "My favorite part is the dessert. Look at the pastry trolley. It's full of all kinds of chocolate treats."

The whole table now began to eye the nearby sweets and I think we were all wishing the sandwiches and toast would get here so that we could move on to those mouthwatering delights.

Just then a man entered the dining room and sat at the table next to ours. All heads turned to look at him and he turned out to be the movie star, Van Johnson. When Cecil went over to take his order, he said that the only thing he wanted was to see the sweets trolley. When it was brought over, to our amazement, he proceeded to ask for every piece of pastry with chocolate in it.

Well, you should have seen our faces. How could anyone be so selfish? Didn't he realize there were other people in the world who loved chocolate, too?

Cecil, seeing the profound disappointment on our faces, came over and assured us that the hotel was well-stocked with other desserts, and he would be sure to bring us their best chocolate concoctions.

We all gave a sigh of relief and I secretly wished that Van Johnson would get really fat and sick from eating all that chocolate.

Over tea, I told everyone that after seeing all those dogs in the park in the morning, I became really lonesome for Muffin.

"Interesting that you should say that, son," my father replied, "because your mother and I were talking about the very same thing the other night. And we've decided to look for a dog for the family. There's a family with Newfoundland puppies in a town a little ways outside of London and we thought the family would take a trip out there next Saturday. We'll see what they have and maybe we'll get ourselves a new dog. Your mother and I miss Muffin, too."

"That would be wonderful," I exclaimed.

I sat back, enjoying the rest of my milk and the delicious chocolate cake Cecil had found for us. But I couldn't wait for the next day when school would start.

The next morning at around eight, my brother and Mr. Lawrence helped me into a small mini-bus that would deliver us to 14 Gloucester Gate on the edge of Regents Park. All ninth graders arrived via public transportation but my father was very nervous about my traveling on the English double-decker buses alone. And of course, as you can imagine, the subways—or as the English called it, the underground or tubes—were out altogether. So he had gotten the school to make an exception and delivery me safely door-to-door with the lower school kids in their small bus.

I felt a surge of energy as I somehow made my way up those four steps to the front door that led to the main hall. I like the way I was dressed, too, in my school uniform of a black blazer and red tie.

Mr. Steven Eckhart, the headmaster, greeted me as I entered. "Albert, I'm pleased to meet you. I hope you will be happy with us."

"Thank you," I replied. "I'm really looking forward to this school year."

The next person I met was Mrs. Helen O'Hear. She was not only my homeroom advisor, but would also be the teacher who would try to teach me algebra as well. I felt lucky to have her, as she was really a wonderful teacher and cute to boot, as was another teacher, Miss Jean Tranoy, who taught me ancient history.

Mrs. O'Hear's homeroom was a short distance from the main door, so I didn't have far to walk. I wasn't sure if my classmates had been told about me in advance or if they were simply used to moving around the world and seeing new and strange people all the time. Whatever it was, the way I walked seemed to make no difference to them and I was warmly accepted into the class by one and all.

This would be my very first experience with changing classes and having different teachers for every subject. Algebra, not my best subject, was scheduled first and was like a continuation of my homeroom, since the majority of the class was made up of ninth graders. Mrs. O'Hear really tried to help me and always allowed me to work at my own pace. When the class ended, we all left the room and headed for another activity. But we would always return to the same homeroom for some of our other classes and at the end of the day. Mrs. O'Hear was very kind and arranged for me to leave my briefcase under her desk so I wouldn't have the added burden of carrying it when dealing with the stairs.

My second period was up a flight of very steep stairs in the school's modest library. I had always loved to read so I quickly volunteered for library duty. Every morning it became my duty to make sure that the library was neat and very appealing. I took great pains to display the latest books the library had gotten and would cut out and display any interesting articles on writers or literature that I found in the daily newspapers. I really enjoyed this period and didn't mind the daily climb up, or the slide down, those very steep stairs. Today it would be a different story. But I hear that the American School in London is a lot bigger today and has moved into a modern building with elevators.

Science, my second least favorite subject, was next. This time I had a male teacher, Mr. Michael Hearth. He was the first since Mr. Larry Johnson back home in the States. He was also the only teacher who was English, as all my other teachers were Americans and, like me, only here for a year or two. Our headmaster, Mr. Eckhart, was an exception, as he lived the life of a permanent expatriate. But back to Mr. Hearth.

Mr. Hearth believed in the old style of teaching and made his students copy words out of a book if they were "bad." I was luckily exempt from having to do this, even when the whole class was being punished. I made a model of the human body for the school's science fair, but that's about all I can remember about my days as a science student. What I do remember most about Mr. Hearth was his musical parodies. One that I remember in particular was on the dangers of smoking done to the tune of "Slaughter on Tenth Avenue."

My next class was English. Our English teacher was Mr. Earl Williams, and he was quite theatrical, doing all kinds of things to make the plays and books we read then—and even now—come alive. The main textbook for the course was a survey of English literature, starting with Beowulf and going up to the twentieth century. I especially enjoyed the way the editors were able to sprinkle in enough history of each period so that you felt you were right there, experiencing events as if they were just happening. I loved reading Chaucer's *Canterbury Tales*, and also literature from the Renaissance, as well as reading the great works of Shakespeare and Christopher Marlowe.

My first introduction to Shakespeare was through his tragedy *Macbeth*. Mr. Williams had us read the whole play out loud in class. I thought I was very smart to practice certain parts the night before so that I had them down pat when I raised my hand to volunteer to do a part in class. I did the part of Macduff's son so well that I was asked to perform it in front of the whole upper school (the ninth to twelfth grades) in morning assembly. I still remember "What is a trader?" and "They kill me, mother. Run away, I pray thee."

But what really made the play come alive was a class field trip to the Old Vic to see it performed by the Royal Shakespeare Company. I was in heaven. Not only was the production wonderful (though in all modesty, I thought I made a better son of Macduff), but being in that historic building made me feel that I was back in the 1600's and that the great bard was about to walk into the theater at any moment. In fact, I felt that way about every theater I entered that year. The whole ambience of the London theater was thrilling to me. The playbills of the shows performed hanging on the walls as you went to your seat, the use of the term "stalls" instead of "orchestra," the tradition of playing "God Save the Queen" at the end of each show (which we sang, along with "The Star-Spangled Banner" each day at school in our daily assembly)—it all made me feel totally connected to English history.

The day I saw *Macbeth* was quite special, for as soon as the play was over, I was rushed down the street to the Royal Festival Hall to hear the American jazz great, Louis Armstrong. How much culture can you get in one day?

In the spring, the family took a weekend trip to Shakespeare's home in Stratford-on-Avon. My mother and I attended a performance of *Measure for Measure*, while my brother and father took in a movie. Despite my disappointment at not seeing *Macbeth* for the second time, I was delighted to be in a place where once again I felt connected to centuries of the English theater tradition.

Our next big English class assignment was to write an entry for the third annual A.S.L. (American School in London) Drama festival. The theme that year was the adaptation of a novel into a dramatic form. Out of all the ninth grade entries, my adaptation of the scene of William Saroyan's history class in his novel *The Human Comedy* was chosen to represent our class in the festival. You can imagine my excitement!

The scene's action takes place during a boring history class, when suddenly one of the students starts talking about noses. The highlight of the scene was when a student says, "The hand is faster than the eye, but only the nose runs." Our class had fun doing the show, but, sadly, we didn't win a prize. Well, that's show biz!

All in all, I truly loved my English class that year during which I was introduced to many wonderful books, perhaps the greatest of which was Alan Paton's *Cry, The Beloved Country*.

The academic life was only part of my day at school. The period after my English class was lunch, and that meant a trip to the basement down some very steep steps. I had no choice but to somehow manage to get down to a lunchroom that didn't serve lunch. Each student had to bring his or her own, although milk was provided by one of the London County councils. By the end of the year I was pretty sick of jelly sandwiches.

After lunch there was a study period and then we had gym. Back then I could run a bit and use my arms, so Coach Warner, our gym teacher, wanted me to participate in all aspects of his sports program. It was fun playing American football in Regent's Park. We were quite a sight for the English people out for their afternoon stroll.

My last class was Ancient History, which was taught by Jean Tranoy. It was a toss-up between her and Helen O'Hear as to who was the best and nicest of all the teachers I've had during my entire school experience. My heart still pounds for Mrs. O'Hear, but Miss Tranoy comes in a close second for she really made history come alive for me, especially when we studied ancient Greece. Not only did we read our textbook, but, like Mr. Williams, who had us read T. H. White's *Once and Future King* so that we could get the flavor of medieval England, Miss Tranoy had us read Homer's *Iliad* and *Odyssey*, along with Mary Renault's modern novels *The King Must Die* and *The Bull from the Sea*. These books tell the story of Theseus, King of Athens, from his boyhood through his later career. We were also told to use our creativity and make a model of the aspect of ancient history that we loved the most. With a little help from Michael, our houseman, I made the figures of Plato and Socrates and showed them having one of their many philosophical discussions.

Again, all my teachers allowed me to work at my own pace. It wasn't until many years later that my mother told me that I had been accepted at the school on a trial basis, but at the end of the first week, my parents got a call from Mr. Eckhart thanking them for sending me to A.S.L.

My name appears several times throughout the 1962 school yearbook, *The Gateway*. In it they said that "probably this year will be most remembered for the beginning of the school newspaper." I was listed as school activities editor.

My writing appeared in *The Gateway* as part of my classmates' overall reflections on what living in London meant to us:

## My Reflections

> With nannies and prams
> Dogs and Lambs
> Regents Park to St. James
> Tower Bridge astride the Thames

I felt very proud to be included amongst the school's talented poets. I also had my ideas incorporated into our class's entry into the school's talent show. I was the new singing sensation—BONY DICE. Needless to say, my singing career only lasted a day and was no real threat to Mr. Chubby Checkers. But I had fun.

Of course school wasn't without its downside. A minor inconvenience was that in December I was still taking the school bus with the lower school kids while all my classmates traveled freely through the London transport system. I felt so left out. But my father wouldn't budge, insisting that I wasn't able to travel on my own in such a big city. I couldn't understand his logic as he seemed to have no problems about my traveling in and out of New York City by myself. Why was London so different? I never found out, but early in January of 1962 he told me that the school had been notified that starting on the 15th of January, their transportation service would no longer be required, and that with my brother's help I would be going to school via the London double deckers.

I was so excited! What a New Year's gift! I not only took the bus, but had to change at Oxford Circus and cross a big street before getting onto my next bus. I was on my way to adulthood.

Soon, traveling around London by myself, or with William, was going well. I had no problems getting on or off the Number 3 or 74 buses, despite the high step up and off. (I don't think I would fare that well today. With the loss of mobility in my right leg, I can no longer lift it as high.) I also managed the English "zebra" crossings, so named for the zebra-looking stripes painted onto the street. There was no button to push that would light up a sign saying "walk," but cars automatically stopped when they saw me enter the zebra area so that I could safely cross the street. Back then, the English played by the rules. I just hope it's the same today.

Anyway, after my first week of commuting by public transportation, my father came to me and said, "I guess we always knew you could do anything you set your mind to. Just never stop standing up for yourself." I thanked my father and hoped in my heart of hearts that this would never change, and I would always be able to not only stand up for myself, but be victorious in all my struggles as well.

Not too long after that, however, my father almost regretted his words of praise. It was on a Saturday night and I had gone to the theater, as I usually did. Only this time, when the performance ended, I couldn't find a bus, and no taxi would stop for me on account of my disability. Cab drivers seeing me for the first time usually assume I'm drunk and don't stop. I didn't know what to do, so I started walking in the direction of home, hoping that along the way I would eventually find a taxi that was willing to stop for me. Well, it was getting late—past eleven, and all London buses stop running after eleven. No cabs were in sight. I started looking for a phone booth so I could call my parents and tell them not to worry, that I was all right. But I couldn't find a phone booth, either. (I later learned that if I had walked down into a subway—the English "underground"—I would have found an abundance of phones.) So I just kept on walking, going through Hyde Park, a few miles down the road.

Around midnight a cab finally stopped for me and brought me safely back to 29 Palace Gate. The driver was wonderful and came upstairs to explain to my parents that a lot of his fellow drivers don't stop for disabled people because they assume that their uneven gait is due to drunkenness.

My parents thanked the driver and then told me that I should have tried harder to find a phone to let them know I was safe.

I felt relieved that they didn't stop me from traveling by myself, for I was sure that the incident would have ended my independence for good. That didn't happen, and by the time the next Saturday rolled around I was back on the street, this time safely in a taxi on my way to Festival Hall to hear the London Symphony play Brahms' Second Piano Concerto. My parents were willing to give me a second chance, but I knew I had to do everything humanly possible to make it home safely. And luckily, I did.

I was still traveling, but now I faced an even bigger journey. It was a journey of a very different kind. One that can go on for a long, long time. A journey that is not easy to end. It is the journey of rejection by someone of the opposite sex.

My first rejection of this kind came when I asked Judi to go with me to the sophomore prom. Up to that time, I had really only had one date, and that was to my eighth grade prom back in America. I'd had a really good time that night, dancing every dance, despite my disability. So when the opportunity came to take a date to another dance, I didn't hesitate and immediately asked Judi Dickson.

There was an advantage of being in a small school. We were invited to all the proms. After all, there were only twenty pupils in each class at A.S.L., and since a big percentage of the students were girls, the dances were open to the entire high school, so the girls could go with boys from other classes.

When I asked Judi to go with me, she gave me a big smile and said, "Thanks, Albert. I'd love to go with you. It's so nice of you to ask me."

She was still smiling when she headed down the hall. As for me, I was not only smiling, too, but I was on cloud nine for the next few hours. Unfortunately, by the end of the day, my smile had turned to a frown, and I even had to fight back tears.

It happened as we were leaving school for the day. Just as I was about to start going down the main staircase, Judi caught up with me.

"Albert," she exclaimed. "Remember how excited I was when you asked me to the dance this morning?"

"Yes," I replied, feeling that what I was about to hear would not be good news. "What's up?"

"Well, I'd never been invited to a dance before you asked me, and now—what do you know—I was just invited again."

"What do you mean?" I asked. "Does that mean you won't be going to the dance with me?"

"I'm afraid so, Albert." There was a pause before she continued. "I was so excited that you had asked me, and I was all set to go with you—but then last period, in study hall, Chuck Anderson passed me a note asking me to go to the dance with him. Here, you can see the note."

She showed me the note and I read: "I want to take you to the Prom. Chuck."

I didn't know what to say.

"I'm sorry," Judi continued. "But I really want to go with Chuck, so I told him yes." She looked at me, and must have seen how upset I was. "But I'll see you at the prom, Albert."

She started walking down the hall and I began my difficult descent down the stairs. Judi's insensitivity upset me terribly, but I was also angry that someone like Chuck, who didn't speak with a stutter, or have any other kind of disability, didn't have the courage to ask Judi to the prom except by giving her a note.

When I got home, my mother asked me how school was that day. Somehow, I was able to say it was great. In my heart, though, I was not only feeling the pain of Judi's rejection but I knew with a chilling certainty that there were going to be many more Judis out there. The future, I feared, was going to hold many days when I would be staying at home instead of being caught up in the fun and excitement of a party. But for now, I was determined to go to the sophomore prom and enjoy it as best I could.

The big night arrived, and dressed in my new blue suit and matching blue tie, I slowly made my way up the front steps leading into the school. All the dances were held in the big auditorium right across from the main entrance to the school.

"Well," I said to myself, "at least I won't have far to walk."

Although I was excited to be at the prom, for I just loved dancing, I was nervous and my stomach was churning. Had I made a mistake coming alone? I wondered. How would I feel when the music started and I didn't have a partner? And how would it be when Judi and I saw each other? But I almost forgot these questions when I heard the music begin, for music has always had the power to fill me with good feelings, and the emotions that melodies aroused in my heart rarely let me feel that I was alone.

In an upbeat mood now, I entered the auditorium and saw people dancing to "Rock Around the Clock." And then I saw Deanne Devoy coming toward me.

"Hi, Albert," she said with a smile. "I see you're here by yourself, too."

"Yes, I am," I replied. "But how come you're here by yourself?"

"Simple," Deanne said. "No one asked me." There was a pause as Deanne studied my face. "You look surprised."

"I am," I replied. "I thought all cute cheerleaders were assured of a date. Doesn't it come with the territory?"

"Not always," she exclaimed. There was another pause. "Well, are we going to stand here all night, Albert, or are you going to ask me to dance?"

The music was starting again, and without another word, I took Deanne and led her onto the dance floor.

Deanne and I had fun that night. We danced practically every dance, including the Lindy. Even though we were just friends, I couldn't help but be taken by that warm smile of hers. And it helped that we were both short, so instead of having to look up at her, I could look straight into her eyes.

During one of our dances, Deanne asked me how I was getting home. I told her that Michael, our houseman, was picking me up at eleven.

"Why don't you call your parents and tell them that my father would be glad to take you home."

"That's nice of you," I said, "but are you sure it's not too far out of the way? After all, I'm on the other side of town from you."

"I know, but that doesn't matter. Don't you remember that my father took you home one night from the theater?"

I remembered very well. It was a night when I was coming out of the Strand Theatre and a man came up to me and asked me if I would like a lift home. I remember hesitating, wondering who this man was and why he was being so kind.

Sensing my uneasiness, the man said, "Don't worry, Albert. You can trust me. I'm Deanne's father."

He did look like a person I could trust, but to be absolutely sure, I had to ask him one more question. "Deanne who?" I said.

"Why, Deanne Devoy," he replied.

That's all I needed to know and I started to walk slowly across the street to the Devoys' car.

Now, at the dance with Deanne, I said, "I'll be right back. I'll just phone my parents. Don't go anywhere."

Soon I was back at Deanne's side. "Mission accomplished," I said.

"Great," Deanne replied. "Now we'll be able to spend more time together."

The music started again, and again I took Deanne's hand and led her onto the dance floor.

We danced the rest of the night. The dance floor was small and very crowded so I couldn't see if Judi was having a good time. But it really didn't matter anymore that she had turned me down. I was sure I was having more fun without her.

Entering the backseat of the Devoys' car, I got a friendly greeting from their small poodle.

"Excited to see Albert again, Franz?" Mr. Devoy asked.

"He seems to remember me," I said.

"He sure does," Mr. Devoy said. "Especially after all the loving you showed him when I took you home the last time. So tell me, Deanne, did you have fun tonight?"

"Oh, yes, Dad," Deanne replied. "It was wonderful."

"So you're glad you listened to your parents and went to the dance."

"Oh yes," came two voices from the backseat.

Arriving at 29 Palace Gate, after giving Deanne a kiss on the cheek and thanking her for a good time, I got out of the car and her father helped me up the stairs that led into our front hall.

Deanne and I remained friends. We never dated, but when it came time for the freshman class to host the spring dance, Deanne and I were a pair. Judi came to the dance, too, but she came alone. I heard that after she had "undated" herself with me at the sophomore prom, she was never asked the another prom again. I don't know what happened, but I like to think that she was being paid back for her insensitivity. To show that there were no hard feelings, however, Deanne allowed her to have one dance with me that night.

I had a great time at the dance, and once again the evening ended with Deanne's father driving me home. Looking back on those days some forty-five years later, I feel a sense of loss at not having gotten to know Deanne better.

At the end of the year, both our families moved back to the States, and we were often in touch by phone and exchanged greeting cards. (I can remember receiving a very racing Halloween card with the salutation, "I want to scare the pants off you!") But the distance between my house in Long Island and her house in New Jersey proved too much for two new sophomores in high school and we soon lost contact. But twelve years ago, after my twentieth high school reunion, I tried in vain to find her. Now, writing this memoir, with the help of modern technology, I once again gave it the old college try. With her brother's and father's first names in hand, I went to my computer where, on the Internet, I have telephone directories from all over the country. I was successful in locating her brother, and contacting him by e-mail, only to learn that Deanne had passed away. I was sad for Deanne and sad for myself, wondering what might have been if I had found her earlier.

So far, I've told you about many aspects of my life that wonderful year in London and about our trips abroad. But I haven't told you yet about the dog, and this story would surely be incomplete without your hearing about the new addition to our family.

Remember how we were all so lonesome for our Newfoundland dog, Muffin? Well, the first weekend after school opened that September, the family took a trip into the English countryside and got another Newfoundland dog. This was my first experience visiting someone who raised dogs for breeding. And strangely enough, the woman who answered the door actually looked like a Newfoundland.

After the hellos were dispensed with, we were taken around back where the puppies awaited adoption. The cries of what I interpreted as "Please take me and give me a good home!" could be heard from miles away. My father wanted a male dog, and my mother wanted a female. She had heard that females were easier to handle. (I wonder if she still thinks that.) A male was finally chosen and my father immediately named him Winston.

Winston was very friendly and playful and the whole family grew to love him. Every morning my brother took him out, sometimes taking him for a walk around Winston Churchill's home. Winston, the dog, was treated like royalty in our home, with his own room and the use of the fire escape to sit out on during the day.

The funny thing was that there was a rule that no pets were allowed in our building, and here we were with this big black dog who would grow to be twenty-eight inches high at the shoulders. Thank goodness for the Englishman's love of dogs, for I don't know how else we could have gotten away with our secret tenant. We were put to the test one day when the owner of our flat, an ambassador from Argentina, flew to London on business and wanted to stop by his home for a visit. Well, you should have seen us rushing Winston into his room and locking the door. We all hoped that he would somehow have the good sense during our landlord's visit not to bark. Luckily, we had gotten the rental office to take an inventory of all the valuables before we moved in and we were able to assure the owner of the flat that we had put most of them in storage for safekeeping. So at least we didn't have to worry about that aspect of the visit. But although we were all very nervous, the visit went well. Our "visitor" was pleased with what he saw and took us at our word that he didn't need to look into the messy room off the fire escape. Somehow I had a feeling that he already knew we had a dog and since he saw nothing amiss in the apartment, he felt there was no need to say anything.

Winston really became a big part of the family that year. My brother walked him in the park every day (or I should say that Winston walked William, as the knees of his pants could attest.) And once in the park, Winston had a ball. He played with every dog he saw, no matter the breed or size. The English just loved Winston. Everyone we met asked to either pet him or ride him. The family's standard reply was, "Winston only gives rides on Tuesdays between three and four." As you can imagine, we always avoided Kensington Gardens on Tuesday afternoons.

Winston also liked watching TV with us and would try to sit on the sofa when he thought his "father" wasn't looking. He would also start to bark whenever there was a sad or violent scene. He especially liked it when the family was all together. I can still remember the times when we would all take the elevator down to go outside. Once we were outside, if I turned right to go toward the shops and he turned left with the rest of the family to go to the park, he would start to whine, obviously upset that I was not going to be with him and the rest of my family.

Winston even enjoyed the family Christmas on the English west coast in Devon. For Christmas that year we visited two sisters my father had met while stationed in Devon during the war. Alice and Sister Dee were two people out of a storybook. Devon was very cold that December. It was so cold in fact that Mother never left her chair near the fire. Dad, William and Winston, on the other hand, enjoyed running along Devon's sandy beach. Alice and I took brisk walks around town.

My father, brother and Winston could be seen running up and down the beach, and it was hard to tell which family member was enjoying himself the most. It's a shame that dogs can't write, for I'm sure Winston would have written a beautiful verse about that bleak gray day when he was jumping around on the beach. To him, the sun must have been shining.

While Winston played on the beach, the rest of us "ran" around the house keeping warm. There was no central heating in the house we had rented, but my body was getting used to the cold so I didn't need to sit right on top of the heater as my mother did. It made me appreciate all the comforts we had back in America. There were some homes in Devon and in other parts of England that didn't even have indoor toilets. (I know this was true in some places in America, but I didn't know that then.)

Despite the chill in and outside the house, the spirits inside each one of us were full of joy. The dining table was set very traditionally, with the very decorative Christmas cracker party favors. The English go to great lengths in decorating each cracker with a festive scene. You can imagine the huge explosion that was heard when all those people seated at the table pulled the strings of our Christmas crackers at the same time!

My prize was a plastic figure of an English bobby. The dinner was being tape recorded, and when played back we all laughed at my mother saying how much she loved the Brussels sprouts, and could she please have seconds and even thirds.

Alice and Sister Dee were typical unmarried women who had grown up in a small town in Devon and lived there until they died. (I heard that Dee did have a brief affair during the Second World War.) It was refreshing to see people living in England in the 1960s who seemed untouched by modern ways. It wouldn't be until 1972 that they would have their own television. But the two sisters were fun to be with and we never got tired of hearing Alice telling stories about her days as a local Brownie Scout leader and of her girls calling her Brown Owl. Their walls were full of holiday cards from all over England. Alice, although uneducated, had a lifetime effect on these young girls. She was like a good teacher one remembers for the rest of one's life.

In the spring we invited the two sisters to visit us in London. Unfortunately, only Alice took us up on our invitation. It seems that she was the more adventurous one, having traveled by bus to Cornwall, a nearby area. Sister Dee, on the other hand, had never left their little village.

The big day arrived and there was Alice dressed in a brand new dress. Well, actually it was an old dress that she hardly ever wore, so it looked new. Alice was quite a sight with her two long gray pigtails rolled over her ears so they looked like earphones. If one didn't know better, one would think she was sent over by central casting to appear in a somewhat weird production of *Alice in Wonderland*.

As you can imagine, she was like a kid in a candy store. She had never seen so many cars on one street. And her eyes and face just shone when my mother took her to watch the Changing of the Guard at Buckingham Palace. She said she could hardly believe that she was seeing this spectacle firsthand. "Oh, thank you, thank you," she kept repeating. "I can't wait to tell Dee."

A funny thing happened when we took Alive to the Savoy Hotel to visit one of our friends from Paris. She walked ahead of us and headed straight for the lifts.

When she got into one of them, she tried in vain to figure out how to start it. She was beginning to be quite upset when an employee of the hotel approached her and asked if he could be of some assistance.

"Yes, you can," Alice replied. "I can't seem to get the lift to work. Can you please show me?"

"Madam," the man said, "you don't have to work the lifts in the Savoy."

Just then we arrived. "What's the problem?" my father asked.

"No problem, sir. I was just explaining to this lady that it isn't necessary to work the lift at the Savoy. We do."

My father thanked the man and we all got into the elevator and were taken up to visit our friend.

The next day we put Alice on the bus that would take her back to Woolacome. She seemed happy during her brief stay with us and I wondered what tales she would tell Sister Dee. I also thought how nice it would be if Sister Dee came for a visit, too. And that did happen about a month before we moved back to the States.

Sister Dee couldn't get used to the sounds of the city of London and couldn't wait to get back to the silence of the Devon coast. To my knowledge, neither Alice nor Sister Dee ever made a return trip to "Foggy London Town."

Speaking of fog, I only really remember a few days of it during my many later years of residence there. Was I in so much of a fog during those years that I missed Mother Nature's vapors? Or did the song and all those movies lie? No matter, I was always wide awake during my time in London, enjoying it to the fullest, no matter what the weather.

But back to Alice and Dee. I was just a young teenager at the time and thought they seemed like they belonged in a fairy tale. But when I was older and spent more time visiting with the sisters, I came to appreciate their simple lifestyle and their wonderful outlook on life. They were still cooking on a wood-burning stove and stored the meat in a room called a "larder." They never purchased a gas or electric stove, or even a refrigerator or freezer.

I learned there and then that some people thought that the sisters were strange, like they think of me as strange, but like Alice and Sister Dee, I've come to ignore them and carry on doing whatever it is I'm doing and find that it all works out in the end. The chicken is just as tasty whether it is cooked on a wood-burning stove or a gas-burning one. I learned an important lesson from my experience with these two sisters: never let other people discourage me from doing things in my own way and at my own speed. And I know that if I failed at a task even though I did the best I could, that maybe that was better than not trying at all. From Alice and Sister Dee I gained peace of mind that has helped me through the many years ahead.

When I was older, and traveled to England to live or visit, I always found time to either call or visit with the sisters.

Another thought about the sisters, and that is how similar they both were to my maternal grandparents. My grandfather was an idealistic lawyer who wanted so much to help people in need of legal advice that if they couldn't pay him, he often accepted payment in the form of barter. Alice and Sister Dee bartered their lives to help others.

I had never seen a year go by as fast as that one. It seemed as though I had just gotten off the airplane that August of 1961 and now it was June of 1962 and time to say good-bye to England and return to the United States.

Life is funny. People were not at all sure how I would manage in England and were glad that I stayed in the states those eight months so I could graduate from eighth grade and attend summer camp. Now, to everyone's surprise, I was the most vocal member of the family in favor of staying in England. I did manage, however, to spend an extra week while the rest of the family, including Winston, were traveling back by boat. I flew back with Michael, our houseman, and met everyone back at our home in Brookville, Long Island.

Seated on the airplane, Michael said, "Look out the window, Albert, and take one last look at London. You might not see it again."

I felt a lump in my throat, for Michael's words had such finality to them. Surely, I told myself, he didn't mean that he thought I'd *never* travel abroad again. I was about to turn sixteen in November and in my mind I planned to do a lot more traveling before my time was up.

Events over the next several months proved that Michael was right for himself, but neither of us knew it at the time.

As we headed out toward Brookville, I found myself filled with so many mixed emotions. Initially I hadn't wanted to go to London and had stayed behind for eight months before joining my family. Now, back home, I wished I were still in London. Deep in my heart, I knew I would return one day.

The first thing I saw when we drove up the driveway was that it was full of packing crates. Then I saw my family who looked rested from their leisurely return by boat. And then—there was Muffin, tail wagging, running to greet me.

I was glad that Muffin was still alive. She was thirteen years old and that's old for a Newfoundland. I felt her bones on the top of her head. She was no longer the young playful dog that used to lick my feet. But at least she was still here.

I learned later that my father found her lying in her favorite spot among the pachysandras. It took her just a few seconds to remember my father's smell, and then it was as though the last eighteen months had never happened.

While this was going on, Winston was still in the car. Since he had quite a reputation as a "ladies' man" around the London parks, I wondered what he would think about Muffin, or what he'd attempt to do. One could only guess.

When Winston was let out of the car, he immediately went over to Muffin, all ready to "introduce" himself. But as he got closer to Muffin, he realized that although Muffin was a lady of the same breed as himself, she was very old. So, believe it or not, he slowed down his pace to an even slower walk, and approached her as he would his own mother. Dad was amused at seeing them both together, and when it came time for dinner, or for them to get a drink of water, Winston would always stay in the background until Muffin was served.

One can never be sure about animals, but I do believe that Muffin enjoyed her new company. But she didn't let anything change, and she was still queen of her own doghouse and continued to be mistress of the grounds. Muffin had the run of the grounds and her dog house was under my parents' window. Winston, on the other hand, had a house in a gated, fenced-in area. I guess my parents were afraid that Winston might run away. My father also sent Winston to dog training school, but Winston never gave up his habit of jumping up on anyone who came near him. My cousin is one of the many people who can attest to his friendliness. There were only two exceptions to this: my mother and myself. I guess since we got Winston when he was a puppy, he had a chance to get used to us and realized that we would each be knocked down if he ever jumped on us.

As for my own adjustment to being back home, I had mixed feelings. I still wished my father had taken that job in Paris and that the family still lived in Europe, but in addition to that, I was anxious about where I would be going to school in the fall. Mr. Eckhart had told my parents that he thought I would do best in a small school like the American School in London. The only small high school in our area, however, was Friends Academy, a private school run by the Quakers. But no one knew if the school would accept me, and if they did, no one knew if the Quakers of Long Island would treat me with the wonderful warmth and understanding that I had experienced in the school in London.

Luckily I had some time before I had to face these questions, for no sooner had I unpacked from London than I had to pack up again—this time for a six-week stay at Homestead Camp.

Homestead Camp was mainly for junior high school students, but I had so much enjoyed my past two summers there that the director tried to come up with some kind of scheme that would allow me to return.

Usually, the kids who wanted to return and were in the tenth grade were offered jobs as junior counselors. But for me, being disabled and still speaking with a terrible stutter, not to mention the trouble I had in navigating the rough terrain that surrounded the camp, no matter how much I wanted it, a junior counselor job was out of the question. So, finally, it was decided that I could return to camp as the assistant to the camp's manager. I would receive no pay, and although the job turned out to be more ceremonial than one of substance, it gave me a taste of reality. For it showed me that despite my many disabilities, eventually I would be able to earn a living. But all that was in the future. For now, I was back at camp, hanging out with a few of my friends for six weeks.

Towards the end of those six weeks I got a call from my mother saying that she and my father had just returned from a meeting with Mr. McNutt, the headmaster of Friends Academy, and that I was accepted into the tenth grade. I would be meeting with Mr. McNutt and a guidance counselor the week I came home from camp.

I was excited now at the prospect of this new school. So far, from early kindergarten through ninth grade, I had always enjoyed the smallness of schools that had no more than one hundred students. This one would also be small, and formal like the American School in London, for all males had to wear a shirt and tie and the females wore nice dresses. I found that I didn't really mind this, for it made me feel quite grown-up.

Mr. McNutt, although a nice person, lacked the warmth of Steven Eckhart. And because the rest of the faculty lacked the enthusiasm of teachers like Helen O'Hear and Jean Tranoy, during my next two years there I felt quite uncreative. The only exception was my English class. My teacher, David Cox, was very interested in the theater and I love hearing the stories of his theater adventures on the Off-Broadway stage. He also had us write a diary. This was the first time I had an opportunity to really write about my emotions, especially the tough ones having to do with my painful feelings of rejection.

I was a teenager and had the same desires of other teenage boys—especially the desire to have a girlfriend. In ninth grade, it wasn't so important. And somehow, being in England, I felt as if I were on a long vacation with so many things to see and do and not enough time. And being an American in a foreign country meant we tended to do most things in groups, so most of the time I didn't feel left out. I remember going to the American Embassy on Friday nights to watch the latest films that came out of Hollywood. These were supposed to be only for the families of the American Embassy and military personnel living in London. A few of the kids in my class belonged to this group and they invited the rest of us to join them on these Friday nights at seven. Afterwards, we'd all go out to a Wimpy (this was in pre-McDonald days). I used to get to the Embassy a little before seven and I'd work my way to the front of the line. At exactly seven, an Embassy guard would open one of the two doors and let me in. After he had seen me safely down the stairs, he would open wide both doors and then what seemed like the whole population of Americans living in London would make a mad dash for the auditorium.

After I left London, I heard that the Embassy staff got stricter and asked to see a special pass that only Embassy and military personnel possessed. But that was later. During my time in London, I could go to the American Embassy to watch a first-run movie with my friends and go out for something to eat with them afterwards. Of course, I'm sure there were times when I was left out of one activity or another, but I was too busy to notice.

Now it was different. I was back in the suburbs of America and there were many weekends when I stayed home alone, wondering why I hadn't been invited to join my classmates in their various after-school activities.

These feelings came even before the school year started. Shortly after I returned from camp I got a call from a Joe Smith, the captain of the Friends Academy's football team, inviting me to join the team. Tryouts would be held the following Friday.

There was a short pause while I was wondering what to say to this Joe Smith. This was the first time in my sixteen years that anyone had asked me to do something I couldn't do. Before, whenever I wanted to participate in sports, the Physical Education teacher always saw to it that I was either the scorekeeper or team manger. This was different. I was being asked to be a player—something I couldn't do.

What should I do?

There was really only one thing I could do, and that was to tell this guy the truth. So, without even a stutter, I said, "I'm very sorry, but I can't play football because I'm disabled. But I would love to come out and cheer the team on."

"Great, Albert," Joe replied. "See you at the opening game."

My mother had been sitting within earshot of the phone. After I hung up, she said, "That was great—the way you handled that."

It wasn't long before I became manager of Friends Academy football, basketball and track teams. Sadly, during my two years the school lacked winning seasons. However, I did get my own byline in the local papers by calling in both the scores and the play-by-play.

My biggest problem at Friends Academy was social. One day I got a call about a party that I wasn't invited to. The caller asked me if I would be so kind as to let her borrow some of my records. Since I wasn't invited I refused her request.

The caller phoned back, this time asking to speak to my mother with the same request. She was very surprised when my mother refused, too. These were painful times. I did manage to have a date for the junior, but not the sophomore, prom, even though I attended both. However, I wasn't invited to either of the before or after parties that accompanied such evenings.

There was one positive thing and that was learning to take the train into the city all by myself to see Broadway shows.

I experienced my first taste of death during this time: my father's uncle, Neil. He got up one morning, showered and shaved; then as he was opening a new pair of underwear, he sat on the bed ready to put them on but instead fell back onto his pillow and went into eternal dreamland. I, too, wish that when my time comes I will dance off the stage just as peacefully as Uncle Neil did.

The next to die was our dog Winston who was hit by the school bus one rainy day. I will always remember all the children wanting to take a ride on him when the family walked in the park in London.

The family got a new dog, Boo Bo. She was a shorthaired Saint Bernard. There weren't anymore Newfoundlands around that could compare to either Muffin or Winston.

Shortly after Halloween, Muffin got sick and died a few days later.

Shortly after Muffin's death the family got a playmate for Boo Bo. Yogi was a wonderful longhaired Saint Bernard and soon the two dogs became inseparable.

Michael left us at this point and was never heard from again.

I knew then that what Michael said to me on the plane coming back from England about not seeing the country again really applied to him and not me. For I was sure as I ever will be that I would see England and the city of London again.

It was during this period, September 1964, that the family moved to Green-wich, Connecticut.

I was about to start my senior year in high school. I was about to give the Greenwich public school system a chance at educating me.

The house was not quite finished when school started so my brother and I were forced to spend the first week in the home of a business associate of my family who had children in the school. The second week we stayed with my grandparents in a local hotel, the Pickwick Arms.

I was terribly worried about how I was going to manage this new school and the whole big situation totally overwhelmed me. The school was just too big and I played hooky. I wanted to give up so I stayed away from school.

It takes three strikes before a person could be called "out." I had only two, or maybe just one, strike against me.

On the Friday of our second week, my parents arrived home from their vacation and the family finally moved into our new home. On the Rocks was spectacular. (Since it was built on a rock foundation, my dad named it "On the Rocks.")

I fell in love with my room immediately. Its oak paneling and large windows gave it the feel of an English sitting room. My desk was placed right under the windows, giving me a wonderful view of both the swimming pool and the lake beyond. I knew that I had to get back to school for this room was just made for studying.

Maybe these last two weeks of despair served as an eye opener to the bigger world that awaited me with all its failings. I knew then that come Monday morning I would be back in school and all would be well.

Monday morning came finding me again back at Greenwich High School, only this time with a less strenuous course load as I only needed nine more credits to graduate. I ended up studying International Relations, Problems of Democracy, and American Literature.

It was then that I decided to take my days at Greenwich High School one step at a time. I was learning that there would be many people throughout my life who would not like me, so I must learn not to run and hide each time someone said something negative to me.

I headed to my first class, International Relations, with a big smile on my face. The teacher, a Mr. Joe Mottolese, was glad to see me. It was arranged with one of my classmates, Randy Peyton, to borrow his notes and get me caught up on the work I had missed. For me, this was the beginning of a lifelong love for anything Asian. I follow international events to this day.

What made this course most gratifying for me, however, were the wonderful friends I made in the class. Besides Randy, there was Alan Bennet, George Faust, Geoff Beal, Sue Gay Johnson and Lynn Slaughter, who sat in the back row. Every morning when she came into class she would catch my eye and would either smile or wave. Little did I know then that Lynn and her husband would turn out to be most special friends during the remainder of my life. I enjoyed many letters, visits to their home and now exchange Christmas and birthday gifts along with e-mails.

I was feeling especially good about myself and about all the friends I was making. However, I still had a severe stutter. Fortunately, GHS provided me with a speech therapist and suddenly my speech began to dramatically improve.

Surprisingly, the key to the improvement came through another medium: the medium of the written word. The therapist had me write short paragraphs about my life and then had me read them aloud. By the end of the year my stuttering had all but disappeared.

Besides Randy and Lynn, there were other people who went beyond the call of duty in befriending me. Linda and later her husband Jeff remain good friends to this day.

But not everything was wonderful that year. Both Boo Bo and Yogi were killed in separate car accidents on the Merrit Parkway. Till this day their deaths remain a mystery and how they got out of their locked yard does, too. We were putting in a swimming pool and maybe one of the workers let them out of their yard.

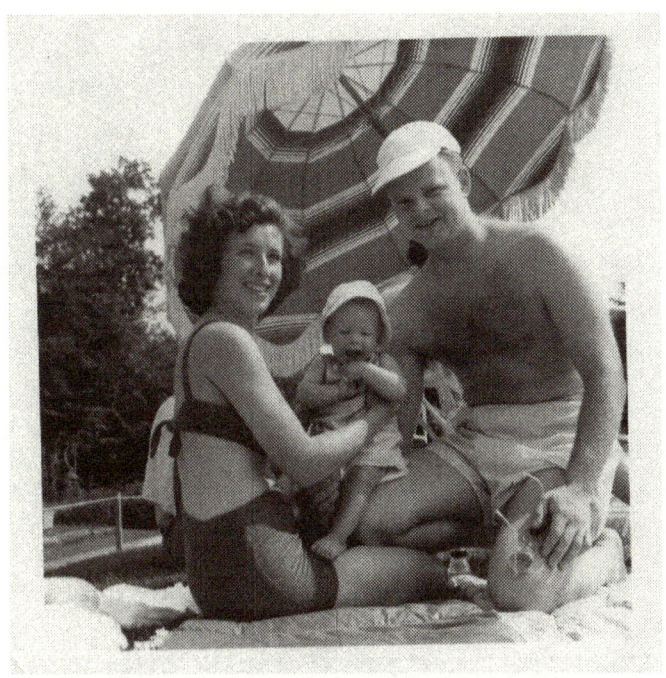

Rea Elias, Albert Elias, and Albert Elias II, 1948

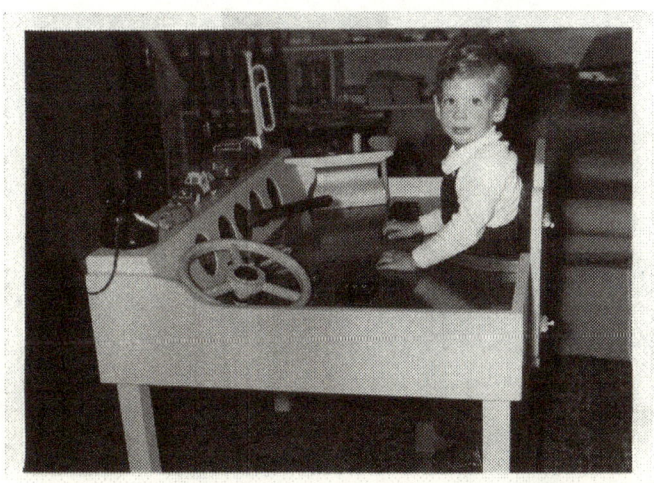

Albert Elias, 1949

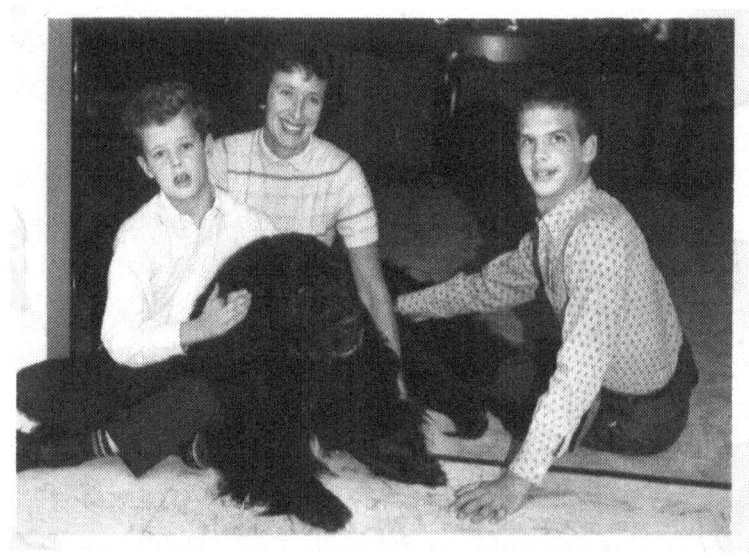

Bill Elias, Rea Elias, and Albert Elias with Muffin, 1959

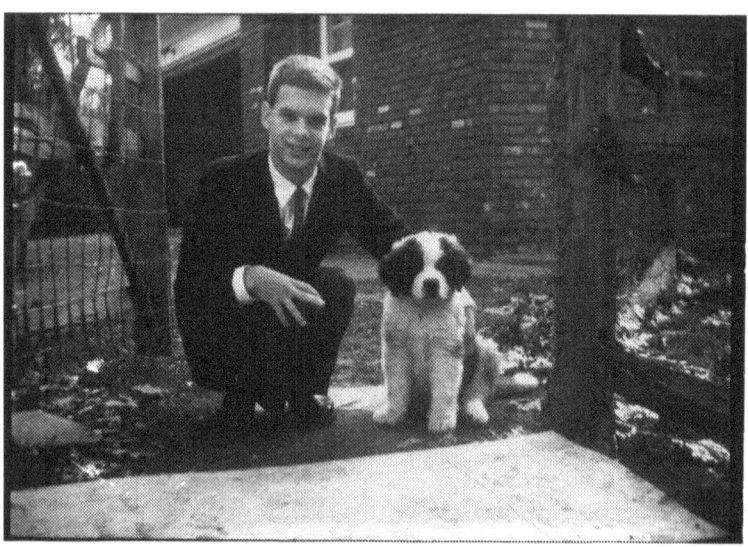

Albert Elias and Yogi, 1959

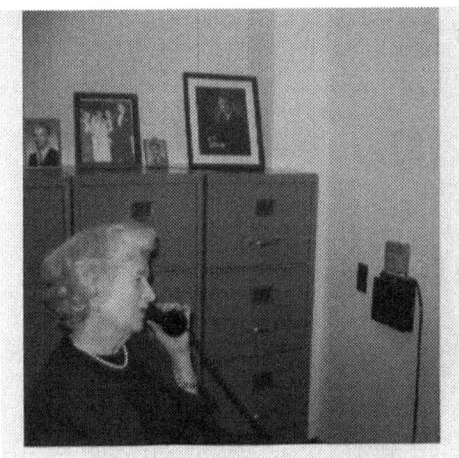

Irene Simon, maternal grandmother

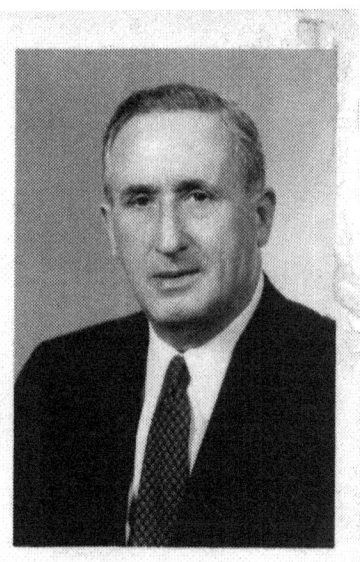

J.I. Simon, maternal grandfather,
December 1962

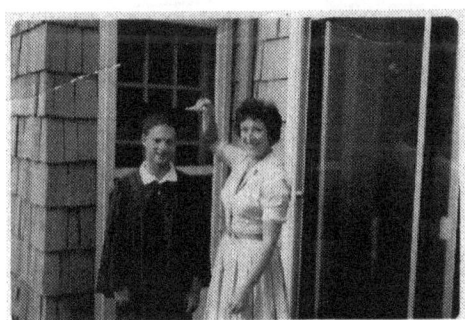

Albert Elias and Rea Elias on high school
graduation day, 1965

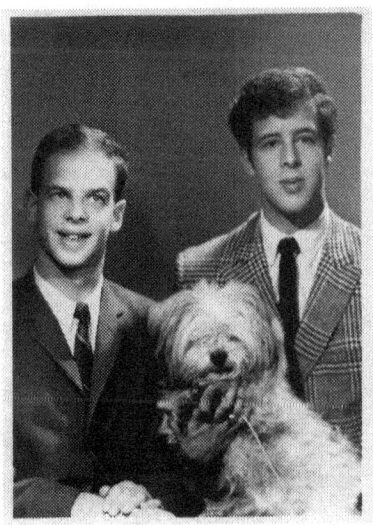

Albert Elias and Bill Elias with
Boozer, 1966

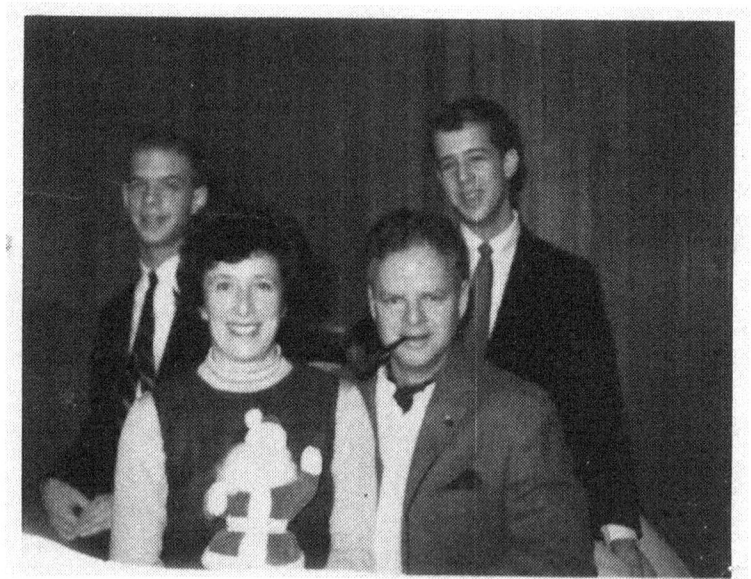

Albert Elias, Rea Elias, Albert Elias II, and Bill Elias, 1966

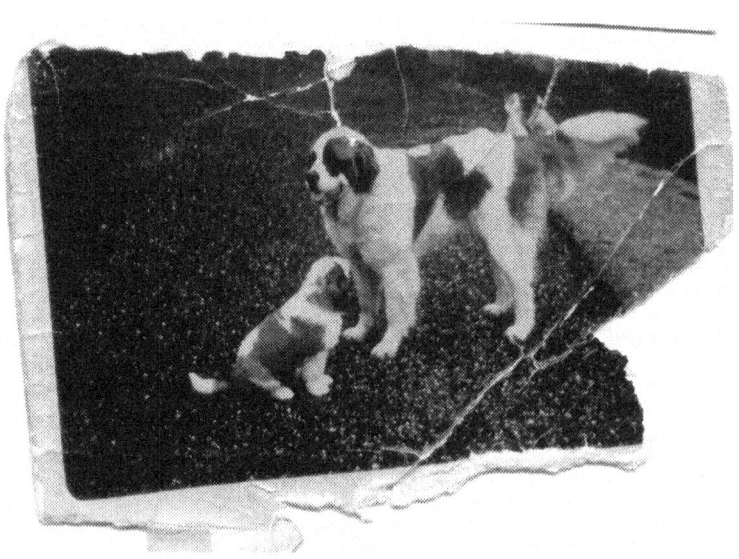

Gloria and Bunkie, 1966

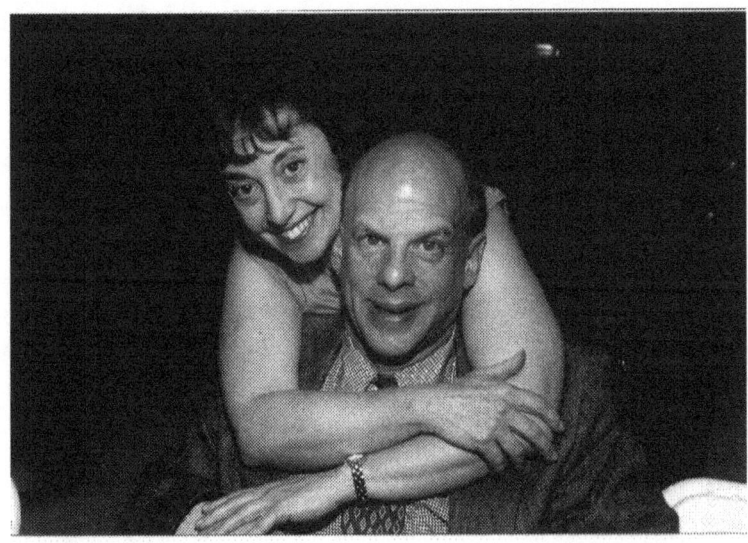

Susan Horowitz and Albert Elias, 2000

The next day the family went out and purchased another Saint Bernard. Gloria was another short-haired who had unusual coloring. But from the very first moment she became my dog. We soon added two more, Muffin II and Bunkie.

Bunkie was male and my parents did not want to mate them. We heard about a new birth control pill just out on the market and decided to give it a try, but the pill killed our dog Muffin. It was decided to get yet another dog, only this time Boozer was a Lhasa Apso.

Unfortunately, as Gloria got older, she developed a form of cancer and died. I was very sad even though by that time I was away at college and living on my own. Bunkie was given away and Boozer died while my parents were in Sanibel and I was living in Scarsdale.

# 2

## The College Years

✦

### 1966–1969

Both my parents wanted me to go to college. But what college? And where? The guidance people at Friends Academy had thought it should be down south in a small school where I wouldn't have to worry about falling on the snow and ice during the winter months. An application was sent to one of the southern colleges where my parents were assured that I would be accepted because the head of the guidance department at Friends Academy was a personal friend of the dean of admissions. The family waited, hoping we would get an answer before moving to Connecticut. No answer came. My father was very upset that he had let a so-called professional do something that really should have been handled by the family. A few years later, a neighbor in Greenwich, whose son attended the college, offered to look into my application and my father's letter that had never been answered, but my father said no, he had taken care of it. I don't know what he found out; it's still a mystery to me why someone would cash a check for the admission deposit and not acknowledge a letter.

Anyway, the family was not stopped from pursuing the college admission goal and after some research American International College in Springfield, Massachusetts was chosen. An interview was set up. There was no application to be made, or money to be paid. That would come later.

The person who interviewed me looked familiar and when he introduced himself, we all said that we had seen him on the baseball diamond as a pitcher for the New York Yankees. My father said later that his arm must have gone bad and that he had apparently decided to take a job in the college's administration office. He also worked in the college physical education department. The interview went well and my parents were pleased at how well I was able to manage the small campus, even though it was not "handicap friendly," but in those days I was much more mobile than I am now. The dorms, however, were another story. They were a good five or six blocks away and in a bad neighborhood. We decided to worry about that when the time came. First I would have to be accepted.

My interview took place over the Christmas holidays and it was not very long afterwards that my parents got a phone call to say that I was accepted. It was a great relief for all of us for it meant that I would be able to continue my education.

The summer before college and after graduation from high school I spent an exciting summer back in Europe along with a two-week visit to Israel and Greece.

I had one memorable adventure in Israel that I would like to share with you. We were told never to wander off by ourselves, especially at night. Did I listen? No! So one night I found myself face to face with an Israeli guard pointing a sub-machine gun in my direction. I noticed he was also carrying a James Bond thriller in his jacket pocket. Although I hoped he was well-trained and would ask questions before doing anything, I felt a chill run through my body and my already-bent knees felt like they were about to buckle. Luckily, he was experienced and could easily see that I was unarmed.

What would happen to my American pioneering spirit if I stopped taking chances?

In mid August I came home, excited by the idea of returning to England when I graduated from college. But that was at least four years away. Now, I had only a little over three weeks to prepare for college and the adventure of independent living.

On the Rocks looked beautiful with all the flowers in bloom, and a swim in the new pool felt so wonderful before breakfast that I was beginning to wonder if it was such a good idea to be so independent so soon. Why not wait a year or so before leaving—with time to enjoy the new house and the Saint Bernards? I was also thinking that it would have been nice if I had spent my junior/senior year at Greenwich High School and my freshman/sophomore years at the American School in London instead of those two years at Friends Academy. Oh well, my parents did the best they could at the time. September 8, 1965, without any more hesitation, I said my good-byes to Bunky, Gloria and Muffin, and getting into a packed car, headed down the driveway towards my new life. But as I left, the three dogs came up to the gate of their yard, as if to say, *Good luck, Albert. We'll miss you.*

Springfield, Massachusetts was a little over two hours from Greenwich by car. As I remember it, American International College's campus was small and its rounded shape reminded me of a fort in the Old West. The only things missing were gates and sleeping accommodations.

My parents wasted no time in saying their good-byes to me. About a half hour after we reached the dorms, they got me unpacked and were on their way home. This pattern of leaving me soon after my arriving at a new place, or furnishing my apartment—all in under an hour—would be something I had to learn to live with for it is something that has never changed. I had to make it on my own.

That first day at college, I felt funny going to the freshman reception alone. Everyone else came with one or two family members. Well, I told myself, I would have to learn to do things on my own. And I would also have to learn to live with a stranger in my dorm room.

Before going away to college, the only real experiences I had of sharing a room with other people was when I lived with the Robinsons for six months before I graduated from eighth grade, and when I went to summer camp. In both cases I knew the people before I shared a room with them. Now, at college, it would be the first time I would be rooming with a total stranger. And I couldn't help wondering how he would feel about sharing a room with a disabled man.

Mark Smith was a junior, but like me, he was new to the school, having transferred from a college in the Midwest. He was also "disabled," but you would never know this unless you lived with him. Mark suffered with ulcers and needed to take medication on a daily basis, and I wondered what could be causing him so much stress and at such an early age. He would spend long hours in the school library, giving me the room practically to myself so that I could either study or listen to my music.

After my parents had left me that Saturday morning to start my new life on my own, I decided to practice walking the six blocks from the dorm to the campus. The college was located in a really blighted section of the state and desperately needed a good urban renewal program. Coming from an upper middle class background, I wasn't prepared for what lay ahead and I found that I was in for an education that went way beyond the college.

I started classes that Monday morning. I would just have to watch myself when I walked through the six blocks. It was really a bad neighborhood.

Again, I thought I would start off slowly by only taking three subjects: Freshman English, Ancient History, and Political Science.

The first month or so went well. I was enjoying my English class and Political Science. Ancient History, on the other hand, was giving me problems. The professor who taught the course didn't take kindly to special students. I found it very hard to transfer out to a fairer professor who was also involved in many humanitarian courses. I would just have to make the best out of a bad situation. I was pleased to hear that the English professor thought I might be the smartest student in the class.

But Springfield, Massachusetts in the mid 60s was not a place for the disabled, or for someone like me who had to spend many hours on his own. There were no theaters or arts of any kind, only urban blight.

The six-block walk was starting to get dangerous, and on many occasions people had to come between me and a group of kids who were chasing me.

The chasing wasn't my only problem. One day I was in the school cafeteria. It was raining heavily and I chanced to look out the window and spotted one of my friends running to get out of the rain. Without hesitating, I went to the back door to let him in. It was really coming down hard, so I opened the door even though the sign said, "Don't Open." I thought it an exception in this case. And besides, I saw many students walk through the door in sunny weather.

Needless to say that my good deed got me reported to the Dean of Students who never let me forget my "bad behavior."

This, however, is not the end of the story. It is now twenty years later and I'm walking down Garth Road in Scarsdale, New York, where I'd just moved. Suddenly out of nowhere the same guy who had reported me to the dean comes up to me and says, "Remember me?" Before I had the chance to answer, he says, "You remember me. I'm the shallow guy from your college days. I hope you haven't run into many more like me."

As he made his way down the road, I yelled, "Thanks for sharing."

I was able to make one friend, David, who ironically came from Stamford, Connecticut, the next town over from Greenwich. I remember one memorable night driving on the Merritt Parkway when a policeman pulled us over and asked us to get out of the car and show IDs. Needless to say, my father had words with this policeman.

David, seeing that I was having problems at American International, told me about Boston University. I told my parents and the transfer was made in time to start my sophomore year.

It's probably only fair to say that American International College wasn't prepared to deal with me and my special needs.

The summer before I was to enter Boston University, my father tried to get me a job with the Unitarian Church at their 25 Beacon Street headquarters. The job fell through. My father contacted a business associate, a Mr. Jack Hausman, to see if he had an opening for me in his textile business for the summer. I worked in the mail room commuting into the city five days a week with my father. It wasn't till I was in my thirties that I would get to know Jack Hausman in his other role as founder of United Cerebral Palsy.

With the summer over I was off to my new adventure at Boston University. I left the dorm, Myles Standish, early so I would have enough time to reach my first class, International Relations. I'm glad that I could still walk the long distances in those days. I eventually ended up with a dual major of government and philosophy. They are two subjects I really enjoy and I have kept up my reading in them till this day.

There was an extra added bonus to my walking to and from the dorm. Often there were people who stopped and talked to me. BU was way ahead of its day and the campus was very accessible for disabled students. The library was nice and quiet for studying, especially on the higher floors.

# Jackie
# From Here to Eternity

I need to take a break to tell of a strange but wonderful phenomenon that happened to me shortly after I entered the university.

It became my habit to study and have my meals in the college library and student union instead of hiding in my dorm. The big reason for this was that it gave me a chance to meet and talk to a wide variety of people and to show them that there was nothing about me that would make them the least bit afraid.

It's very hard for me to carry a tray so I always asked the person directly behind me if they wouldn't mind giving me a hand by taking my tray to the nearest table for me. I usually managed to find a friendly soul to help and even on occasions to sit down next to me for a friendly chat.

This time, however, it was different. A tall blonde woman had taken my tray without being asked and proceeded to take it to the checkout counter and to a table. She shortly returned with her own tray and sat down next to me. This woman knew my name as she called me Albert.

We talked for a while and started meeting regularly for meals. It seemed as though whatever subject came up we both had something to say on it. It was wonderful and it seemed that we were very comfortable with one another, too. There was a certain mood and atmosphere created that made me feel that I never cared if I was with anyone else again as long as I lived.

It's true that she was beautiful and might have made a good model, but that wasn't the reason I found her attractive. No, it was her soul. We were and I think still are soul mates even though many years have gone by since we last set eyes on one another.

There has been no one else in my fifty-nine years that I have shared more with or felt as comfortable just being around or thinking about.

It's wonderful when you can share your innermost thoughts and feelings with another person.

I still harbor warm thoughts and feelings for Jackie even to this day. Like Viktor Frank (whom I mention in the preface to this book), I too have developed an inner life by actively reliving in my mind the happy times and feelings I felt by just being around Jackie.

My imagination has helped keep Jackie alive and fresh in my heart of hearts. I know we will remain soul mates forever.

So, Jackie, in the words of an old Frank Sinatra song: "Sleep Warm! Sleep Well! Sleep Warm!"

Meanwhile, back at Boston University, my life seemed to be going well. I loved my classes, and the independent life that I was creating for myself made me feel very grown-up. My own apartment…would it be next? I thought I would run the idea by my mother to see what she thought. To my relief, she said yes, but that I would have to do the looking by myself.

It didn't take long before I found a nice agent who told me to be at his office Monday morning as he might have just the place I'm looking for, close to shopping and to the university. I couldn't wait for Monday to come.

I fell in love with 15 Keswick Street. I was only five short blocks from campus and there was even a tree growing in front of my window. Plus there was an MTA station and every shop I would ever need only a block away.

I decided to go back to the real estate office and phone my mother with the news. I was not yet twenty-one, so a parent's signature was needed on any paperwork.

My mother was surprised that I was able to find a place so fast and told the nice real estate agent that she needed to first speak to her husband and would get back to him.

The deal was signed within the week and on April 1, 1967 I moved in to my first apartment. I stayed there until I graduated from Boston University in August of 1969.

I managed to get furniture from a neighbor of my parents. It was only on a loan as the furniture would be returned just in time for my parents' friends' own children to use when they entered college.

I managed to get out of my dorm contract with some money back.

After moving in, I got friendly with the manager of the local grocery store who was more than happy to have one of his staff help me home with my purchases. I was very pleased with the extra help and for the manager's offering it without being asked to do so.

It was my first experience with having my own telephone, too. I just loved the number the phone company gave me: 0077. I made the big mistake of putting the number in the phone book. I never did again and even till this day you will not find me listed in any phone directory.

As for my laundry, I found a Chinese laundry at the end of the street and faithfully dropped off and picked up laundry every Saturday. I continued this practice well into the 1990s when the same person who cleaned my apartment began cleaning my clothes.

I felt Mr. Friedrich Nietzsche would have been proud of me: I felt like his superman gaining my own will to power.

My maternal grandparents came to visit my studio apartment quite often. I would sleep on the floor, giving them my bed. My grandfather was able to get the garbage picked up instead of having it sit in the hallway for long periods of time. It saved me from purchasing air freshener every week.

The main door, however, remained unlocked due to the fact that another tenant forgot his key and broke the side window and unlocked the door. The window was never fixed as the landlord refused to repair it.

Time passed quickly. Months turned into years. When I wasn't studying or talking with Jackie, one could find me at Symphony Hall listening to the Boston Symphony. Music helps me create.

A big aspect of my life in Boston was to show the skeptics that I could manage very nicely on my own. I passed the test with flying colors. I guess it was the biggest test of all.

Shortly before graduation, I received the sad news that my grandfather was dying of leukemia. It was sad that the one man who fought so hard for me all my life and wanted me so much to have the experience of college life would not be around to see me walk down the victory mile.

Now, some thirty-five years later, I still get very emotional just thinking that he wasn't there in person, only in spirit.

As graduation came near, I got some bad news from the university as well. When I first arrived at Boston University my father wrote to the geology department explaining my situation and the professor agreed to excuse me from the lab part of the course and I would concentrate my efforts on the non-lab part of any science course. Due to cerebral palsy, my hand-to-eye coordination isn't perfect. Back in 1969, using my left and right hands together was simply out of the question. For some reason, however, the professor who spoke to my dad three years before suddenly changed his mind when it came time to take his course and said I needed the full science course, going back on his word. How was I going to satisfy the lab science requirement that would enable me to graduate?

Leaving his office, I luckily ran into Professor Norbert Kimball, the chair of the philosophy department. He helped me draft a petition that would substitute the Philosophy of Science for Introduction to Geology. He signed it *NHK*. The petition was granted. I sent the signed petition to my grandfather who stayed alive just long enough to read it and know I would receive my B.A. on August 15, 1969. My mother and both grandmothers witnessed the graduation.

At graduation I kept looking for my dad but he wasn't there. The two men who had made this day possible were absent. One was dead. But where was the other?

Someone told me later that my dad didn't come because he was so upset over the hard life that that dice had dealt me that he just chose to be absent. But I didn't understand that. I had won this round! He should have been proud that he had instilled in me the strength to persevere against all odds and still reach my goals.

I got in line to receive my diploma. The line was moving rather fast and the graduates were descending the stage from both the right and left staircases. I suddenly realized that when my turn came, I would be leaving via the right staircase, with the handrail on the right. That was the wrong one for me. I could only balance myself by holding on with my left hand. What was I going to do?

Looking over my fellow graduates, I didn't see a soul I recognized so, without hesitating, I crossed over to the left side of the stage and down the left staircase. The orderly procession was momentarily disrupted.

I walked out of the auditorium and into the warm August sun with a big smile on my face.

# 3

## *Work*

## Part A
## August 1969–March 31, 1971
## New York City

When I arrived back in Greenwich, there was no clear idea where my life was headed. I managed to obtain a degree from one of the largest universities on the East Coast and seemed to manage my daily living there quite well. Could I do even better? I was over twenty-one, a young adult. Back in college everyone remarked that I possessed excellent communication skills. I was confident that I would find a position somewhere, soon.

For the moment, however, it was decided that I would travel back to Pittsburgh with my grandmother and keep her company while she went through and cleaned up my grandfather's affairs. There would be plenty of time to decide what to do with the rest of my life.

When we arrived in Pittsburgh and my grandfather's office, the first thing that needed to be done was to make some sense out of his unique filing system. Each file was numbered according to some aspect of each individual's personal life. For example, my file was number 15 since I lived at 15 Keswick Street.

After sorting out the files, my grandmother had to deal with the clients. Sadly, my grandfather didn't train another lawyer to take his place after his death so as a result people were unaware of his special ways. He never sent out bills. The lawyers who took over his practice did. My grandmother received many calls from clients who cried on her shoulder. But there was nothing she could do.

The high point for me during this sad time was getting up early and catching the 8:30 bus that took us downtown. I was mixing with the workforce. We saw some of the same faces every morning and that proved exciting to me.

It was also exciting to me to walk into an office building and take the elevator to Grandpa's office which was located on the ninth floor. I practiced my typing skills on the office electric typewriter. It was a big change from the manual typewriter I had used up until then.

During the third week of my stay, my parents phoned to say that they had spoken with the president of Warwick & Legler, an advertising agency that handled my father's business. They were willing to give me a job in the media department doing media expenditure analysis. I took them up on the offer and decided to live at home in Connecticut and commute into New York.

On September 15, 1969, I started my first job. Walking up the front steps of the Seagram Building I was filled with a new burst of confidence. No one would ever question my abilities again.

Mr. John Meskil met me at the elevator and took me to my new office where a desk and electric typewriter were awaiting me. I also was introduced to my immediate supervisor, and to Cynthia and Janet, the two women with whom I would be sharing the office.

Janet was a cute blonde who wore micro mini-skirts. She was very friendly.

Cynthia and I became good friends and still exchange Christmas cards till this day.

My office was located on the 24th floor and had floor-length windows which gave me a spectacular view of Park Avenue down to the Pan American building.

My initiation into the world of advertising came via a study of media expenditures of feminine hygiene products.

In the 1970s it was taboo to advertise these products on television so my study was restricted to the print media.

I did see how some products used TV and recorded expenses both for national and spot TV.

These figures were only estimates and didn't really reflect deals done "under the table."

It was fun being a commuter. I went into work every day on the 7:10 train and came home on the 5:47. When I was leaving Grand Central Station on my way to 52nd and Park, where the Seagram building was located, I first had to take the escalator up into the Pan American building, walk through the building and exit onto Park Avenue where I had a few short blocks to walk until I reached the Seagram building. The way back down into Grand Central Station, however, was difficult. But by asking, I always found a willing arm to balance my descent.

These were fun times, as I just love adventure of any kind, but something inside me told me that my Greenwich/New York City days wouldn't last and that it would not be long before I started a new adventure far away from home. I would be returning to England to live and work.

My father contacted Mr. Norman B. Norman, another business associate, about working in his London advertising agency.

I couldn't wait to hear, as I longed to be back in London. But it was during this time period that England was experiencing one of its many strikes. The postal union decided to go out on strike. Private messenger services were being used to carry the mail all over England and Europe. The overseas mail was terribly delayed. I had to wait three months.

It was the first week in March, 1971. My father got a call from Mr. Norman B. Norman stating that my working papers had finally arrived and that if I so desired, I could start my new life in London as of April 1.

I left Warwick & Legler March 21, promising to keep them informed of my doings abroad.

# Part B
# England: Norman, Craig and Kummel
# April 1, 1971–August 15, 1974

My family was able to contact a friend who lived in London and through her I was able to find me a bed-sit, one room, just like I had during my college days in Boston. I could have it for the month of April and then move into a bigger place in May. The first place was located in Swiss Cottage and the second in Hampstead. Both were very near to where my office was located in Camden Town. It would be a touch of working-class London during my time in Swiss Cottage as each room had a coin-operated electric meter.

During my six years in London, I would come to appreciate the simple things that we in America take so much for granted. Some places in England even lack indoor plumbing. I would get involved with an organization fighting for the homeless. Some say that I was an inspiration to the people working there, not only because of my disability but that someone in my social class would take such an interest in homelessness issues.

I enjoyed my time in Swiss Cottage hearing the noise of the London buses, the diesel-run taxicabs, and the milk floats that brought me two fresh pints of skim milk every morning.

I made friends with a pair of my neighbors. I met them one Friday night. I didn't have a television and needed something to do, so I went and knocked on their door to introduce myself. The door was opened by a woman dressed only in shorts with nothing on top. The topless look was kinda pleasant. She ushered me into the living room to meet her husband, who was fully dressed. After giving me a glass of wine, she sat down on the coach next to her husband. It proved to be the craziest evening I think I ever spent.

It was at this time also that I arranged with the milk delivery float to pay my bills when we saw each other instead of me having to come down the stairs to pay every Saturday. This practice continued in my new flat in Hampstead.

My new apartment (flat) was located on a quiet tree-lined street in Hampstead not too far from Hampstead Heath. I ended up walking through it almost every Sunday watching people fly their many-colored kites.

My office in Greater London House was very different from the one I had at the Seagram Building. The building used to be the Blackcat cigarette factory before it was converted into office space. Norman, Craig and Kummel (NCK) occupied the whole third floor.

I was walking in those days and took the stairs instead of the lift (the word for elevator in England). The back stairs proved to be less steep so I used those. The only obstacle I would encounter would be a group of homeless men.

I was generally ignored despite my vulnerable appearance. I only had one encounter with one of the men and that turned out to be a nice one.

I was coming out of one of the buildings one day on my way to lunch when I fell. One of the older homeless men came over to me holding a cane in mid air. Reaching me, he lowered the cane and stretched out his other hand so that I could easily take hold of it. He helped me get up and gave me the cane. "Here," he said. "Take my cane. I've been living on the streets for some thirty years and as you can see, I'm an old man. You're young and I think a cane would help you walk better." I did take the man's cane and headed for the pub.

The English pub life proved very enjoyable. It was the only place where an outsider could really get a feel for the community. I learned to play darts. My drinks started with light ale, then sherry, red wine, until I finally settled on dry white wine, a drink that I still enjoy today. I remember a great bachelor party. NCK handled the advertising for London Rubber Co., which was the manufacturer of condoms. I remember one of the guys getting hold of a doctor's black bag and filling it with condoms, as well as a user's manual. Those were fun days.

I was soon given a new job at NCK, that of information officer. The only problem was that I had to change offices. Since arriving at NCK, media was the game, just as in New York. I had my own office looking out at the chimneys of northern London. It reminded me of when I was thirteen and had a similar view out of my parents' kitchen window, only then it was of west London. But I was about to say good-bye to the media department and enter the world of marketing. No more private office with a view. A glass partition was the only thing that separated me and another person from the marketing director, a Mr. Richard Ellis. I became lifelong friends with my coworker, a woman named Candis, though everyone called her Candy. She was also an American, coming from Chicago. She married an Englishman. I soon was invited to their home for dinner and the three of us have remained friends ever since.

I was soon going through the daily papers and magazines clipping out articles that I thought would be interesting to NCK's clients and account people.

The *Financial Times* also had their own library on call that stayed open until ten at night, five days a week. I used the service quite often. I can remember one of the clients heard of a product manufactured way back in 1905 and needed to find out the name. It only took one call to the *Financial Times* library to get the answer.

The British papers also had their funny side. The *Sun* always ran a picture of a partially nude woman on page three. And they did carry some articles I was able to use for marketing.

Along with the daily papers, I also had to glean information from magazines. These were mostly in the form of competitive advertising.

There were, of course, the various articles from specialty magazines, like *Forestry* which luckily ran a big spread on chainsaws just at the time when our office in Denmark was making a pitch for a chainsaw company and needed all the information I could find on the subject for the UK market.

My new apartment on Parliament Hill was great despite being on the English "first" floor. People soon got used to seeing me sliding down the stairs.

The apartment didn't come with a TV or stereo. I had brought my stereo and records from America. But not a TV. The Griffins, friends of my parents, who had been so helpful already, were helpful yet again and told me to rent a TV and obtain a TV license. Since the BBC was commercial free, they had to pay for the programs somehow.

The stereo had to wait to be installed, but I finally got ahold of two guys who loved working on Yankee stereo sets. I was all set.

When I wasn't busy listening to music on the weekends, I was busy traveling. Kent, the garden spot of England, was one of my hangouts. I loved to spend the night with some friends of my family on their farm.

Rye, in Sussex, was another place I enjoyed visiting. I stayed in a bed and breakfast run by a couple who used to be in the advertising business. I used to get a kick out of the fact that there weren't any room keys. I wonder if the same holds true today? There was also an old inn in the town that was built in the 1400s. It was on a cobblestone street and was still in business. They served a great lunch.

Stratford-upon-Avon was another stomping ground. I spent the weekend and went to two Shakespearean plays, and had a nice pub dinner at a restaurant called The Dirty Duck. I got a kick out of the fact that a lot of the actors ate there after the performances.

I was walking in those days, not like today when a wheelchair or walker has to be my traveling companion. I remember one night asking a young couple directions and before I knew it, we were having a drink in a local pub. Their kindness didn't stop there as they insisted that on my next trip to Stratford I stay with them instead of the bed and breakfast. I took them up on their generous offer and got to meet their three teenage daughters. A few weeks later I was able to return their kindness and invited the couple to my apartment to spend a long weekend.

They were never in a big city before, so I was more than happy to show them the sights of London.

Life at NCK was beginning to change. The top management, the team that ran NCK's London office, left, and with them went several blue chip clients. I got a quick course on the "other facts of life": no matter how well you perform, it still comes down to who you know. It took a little time to put NCK back together again and the new management team hired all new faces. I sadly said my good-byes on August 15, 1974. The creative team made me a nice card featuring the Albert Memorial, which everyone signed. I still have it today. Along with the friendship of Stan Woodcock-Jones and family and with Simon and Candis Waldram.

Stan is in his 70s now and his eyes are a little weaker, but during my days with NCK I used to visit his country home and enjoyed my time with his wife Terry and their children. We still exchange Christmas cards and e-mails.

# Part C
# Shelter
# September 1974–October 1976

After I left NCK I needed something to occupy my time between nine to five, five days a week. Productive work was important and being part of society at large was important, too. I loved being out there and seeing what everyone was doing, even though oftentimes I was excluded. I still had my vivid imagination and the ability to enjoy the small pleasures that came my way.

My parents did their best to find me a well-paying job. I interviewed with a blue chip pharmaceutical firm and even though I found the work exciting, I found the commute to be terrible. I would have to change buses three different times and, to top it off, I would be paid an English salary with all those taxes thrown in.

I decided that even though the prospect of making money sounded great, it wouldn't really amount to very much once you factored in transportation and the heavy English tax. (At NCK I was being paid in America, where I avoided the English tax and only had Social Security taken out of my salary.) I thanked the people for their efforts and headed to a non-paying job at Shelter. I was already doing work for the organization on a volunteer basis every Wednesday evening and found the commute to be easier. It was also near the Northern Line on the subway (underground) route, which suited me fine, since it was very near my home. The one big advantage of Shelter's location was that it was located in the heart of the theater district. I could work late at the office when I went to shows by myself, or I could leave work only a bit later if I was meeting someone for dinner, without having to worry about fighting the crowds at rush hour. Now I could take my time.

I approached the people at Shelter, The National Campaign for the Homeless. At first they didn't know how I would fit in. They didn't have any other disabled staff members and the doctor they consulted wasn't too keen on the idea, having some preconceived notions about the state of disabled people's physical and emotional capacities. Luckily, the person on Shelter's staff to whom he spoke knew me from Wednesday evenings and just said to the doctor, "Thank you for your input, but we are used to him." Even though I thanked the person for standing up for me, I still didn't have a full-time job.

I decided to stay and hoped for the best. Maybe something permanent would develop if I really showed off my skills. Well, I did just that and it wasn't long before I was happy to be offered a permanent position, even if it wasn't a paying one. At least I would be working five days a week in a field that dealt with people instead of things. I found my niche selling Shelter's many publications.

I stayed at work late, sometimes not leaving Shelter's office before 7:30. Having volunteered on Wednesday nights, I was well aware that the main entrance to the building was closed at 7:00 P.M. and the only way out was through the basement of the next building. Many people thought I was crazy to walk through a dark, empty basement by myself, but I was determined not to let anyone or anything stop me, not even a dark basement.

All this talk about poverty and the world around me was so exciting that I soon forgot that I wasn't being paid or considered part of the staff—even though I was treated as such by everyone except top management.

This was especially true of Les Burrows. I remember working late one night when the phone rang. Sometimes it was from a person needing emergency help, but on this particular occasion, the voice on the other end of the line was a very upset woman looking for her husband, Les Burrows. I had heard his name mentioned several times but hadn't met him. I thought for a moment before answering, and then said that he wasn't at the office, but he might be around the corner at one of the two pubs we all frequented at lunch or after work. "I'll phone around to see if I can find him and have him phone home." She thanked me and I started calling. I got lucky on the second call. Les was indeed there and would phone his wife right away. He thanked me and promised to stop downstairs at the Shelter office and introduce himself the next day. The experience showed people that, given a chance, I could provide a valuable service. I not only gained the respect and trust of someone, but I made two long-time friends. After that night, I had a drink with Les and was invited to dinner to meet his wife. We also went to the theater and spent many enjoyable evenings together. The three of us are still in touch today.

A similar incident occurred shortly afterwards that enabled me to make another friend. It did not last as long as the first, but still was worthwhile. Stu was the photographer for Shelter. It was his job to get photos that the organization used in their publications and fundraising material. One day he was shooting in a slum area up in the northern part of England when he noticed a group of kids hanging around his car. He had notified the police earlier what he was doing, and the make and model of his car, but unfortunately there were no policemen around so, sadly, he could only watch as the kids broke into his car and took his belongings. All his expensive cameras and other equipment were gone. The kids were "kind" enough to leave his sports coat, his wallet minus the cash, and his credit card. I could only guess that the kids didn't know what a credit card was for, or how it was used. It was a good thing because otherwise I don't know how Stu would have managed to get home. Anyway, shortly afterwards, he phoned me and explained what had happened and would I be so kind as to phone his wife. He had been unsuccessful in reaching her. I should just tell her that his plans had changed and that he was on his way home earlier than he had planned. Under no circumstances was I to tell her what had happened. I said I understood, even though I wanted to share the news.

Shortly after Stu's call, I managed to get through to his wife. She was excited to hear the news, as it seems they had had a little disagreement over the phone the night before and it had not been resolved. I wasn't about to tell her the real reason for his early return, but whatever the disagreement was, it was quickly resolved as shortly after that I was taken out for a nice thank-you dinner. Unfortunately, I lost contact with them over the years.

Through those friendships I was starting to learn the business of Shelter and was able to talk to visitors when they came into the office to look over the publications the organization published. Sometimes I made a real impression and was given extra money for the organization's work. Even though I wasn't considered staff, the top management had to notice my contribution as the increased sales from publications soon showed up on the weekly financial statements.

My job expanded when both Stu and Les told me about what they did and I was given the job of fielding their phone calls when they were out of the office.

But no matter what I did, the top management, for some reason, never truly accepted me as part of the staff. Why they were so closed-minded instead of seeing for themselves what a disabled person could really contribute, I could only guess.

I really started to appreciate what the campaign was trying to do when I started selling their publication *Tide Accommodation*, about the problems that arise when people no longer have a job and are forced to give up the home that came with the job. This really hurt the people who worked on farms, the church and other places. Where were they to go? It was bad enough to lose your job, but to lose your home as well was a double blow. I was glad that Shelter was bringing these problems to the public's attention.

Bed and Breakfast Accommodations was another big campaign that got my adrenaline going. It seems that the homeless were being put in bed and breakfast hotels by the local government to get them off the street at night. One might think at first what a great idea, for after all, most English people used bed and breakfast hotels when they went on holiday. They were cheap, as these hotels only provided bed and breakfast, but the rest of the day a person had to fend for himself. When one is on vacation, he doesn't mind because that's what vacations are for: relaxation and doing as one pleases. But this was not the case with the homeless, for after breakfast, which might consist of a bowl of cereal and coffee, the homeless were thrown back into the "cold" street to fend for themselves until nightfall when they were once again admitted back into the hotel for another night. This was defeating the purpose since not only were these people homeless, they were unemployed as well. Where were they to go, and what could they do with themselves all day?

I really worked hard in pushing Shelter's Bed and Breakfast publication. But even though the publications were sent free of charge to local government officials, sadly, they never read them.

Les was very pleased with my attitude as I came from the upper middle class but worried more about people from a lower strata. He said he wished there were more people like me.

Shelter had other publications, on empty property and the newly passed rent act. But the one I remember the most was one they did on redlining. It seemed that the banks would draw an imaginary red line around an area of the city that it refused to lend money in. This, of course, is illegal, and Shelter, with the publication of their findings, really got on the backs of the insurance companies and banks. My phone started ringing off the wall from the moment I entered the office. I had never experienced such controversy.

The top management wanted to get rid of me and started to look for ways to replace me: just as I was finding my niche and learning about the many problems people faced just to secure one of the basics, shelter.

I couldn't really understand this as the publication department was seeing a profit for the first time. And I recorded all of the monies received from over-the-counter sales.

I must say this for Les: he did speak to Chris, the deputy director, who was able to postpone my departure for another couple of months.

My reprieve only lasted two months, however, as Chris left and with him went my last hope of survival with Shelter. Even though I wasn't part of the staff in their eyes, I felt that I was and gained an appreciation for life and for what I was given that has stayed with me forever. I hope that I helped in my own small way.

In the meantime, I had just purchased a new apartment that I sadly had to sell after only two years. I was really enjoying the garden, as the English summer was hotter than usual that year. I was getting used to the three flights of stairs and the walk to and from the train station. I really didn't want to leave London.

I needed to take some time and travel around the good old US of A and see what options were open to me back home as I could not find another job in London.

My brother was about to be married in Toronto, so why not start in Canada? I started to plan a little trip after Toronto. I would be off to Vancouver, also in Canada. Here I could kill two birds: one was to go to an international Habitat conference run by the United Nations, the findings of which I could report back to the people in England. The other was to expand my knowledge and see if Vancouver could be a place where I might want to settle in. After all, it was still pretty wild up there. Maybe after urban life, I might be ready for a bit of the country again.

After Canada, I would go on to Chicago, where the sidewalks might be too steep for me, but it would be fun to see. St. Louis would be next, where I could visit with my old junior high school friend Paul and his family. Then I would head on to Atlanta where a family friend had lined up a job interview for me. I might be getting back into the advertising business there. It was a prospect that excited me, for it had been two long years without a paycheck and although I found the job that I created at Shelter to be interesting and satisfying, it didn't pay the bills and life was beginning to become expensive. I had to get a job that paid. I was also interested in seeing Atlanta.

Washington, D.C. was my next stop. I hadn't been in the nation's capital since seventh grade and had fond memories of the place. Boston is where I would spend the Fourth of July and see a Red Sox baseball game. In the five years I had been in England, I hadn't seen a baseball or American football game and missed the action of both very much. I guess for me, what was going on at Shelter and with the British economy was all for the best for I was beginning to get really homesick for America.

Connecticut would be my last stop. There, I would spend a few relaxing days with my family before heading back to England where I would wait out the sale of my apartment. Too bad I couldn't pack up the apartment and ship it back to America with me. I liked living in London and really didn't want to leave. Besides, thirty was far too young for retirement.

On June 1 I left London for Canada and America, and I had a wonderful six weeks of traveling around. Now it was over and Boston was my choice. Was it the right choice?

I returned to London a few days later, half wanting to stay but knowing deep in my heart that my days there were numbered.

Nevertheless, I was glad to be back. England in mid-July, as I've said, was warm and stayed light till around 10:00 P.M. The people at Shelter were glad to see me, offering me my old job back. They weren't able to find a replacement in the six weeks I was away.

I sold my apartment to someone from Shelter and planned to leave England for good November 1.

I spent my last days in London working and going to the theater. I also traveled to parts of England that I'd missed. A five-day trip to Edinburgh, Scotland, was among the highlights of my travels.

Shelter had moved their offices very close to the old Vic Theatre and Royal Festival Hall. This was a good location for me except for the subway.

The nearest subway stop to Shelter's office wasn't very handicap friendly. The station wasn't deep enough for a proper lift, so I was forced to use the escalator, which turned out to be too fast. One day I got my shoe caught and even had my shoe come off. I remember being in some pain and almost crying when a kind person behind me yelled to the subway staff to turn off the machine as someone was in trouble. From that day on, I always traveled with someone, usually Les, who would take me down to the Northern Line platform and then take the escalator again, this time heading toward the Southern Line platform and home. I even wrote to an organization that was established to help the handicapped to advise them about the problem this kind of situation posed for me and for others. Les got a kick out of my calling the others "all the Alberts of the world."

Sadly, the organization was not much help. They expressed sympathy and wished me well in my fight, but escalators remained a problem for a lot of disabled people.

# Part D
# The American/English Life
# April 1971–November 1976

Before I leave the wonderful British Isles, I thought I'd tell you a little bit about my everyday life outside of work and about a few of the people I met and the various places I visited.

I was only on the job for a week when the English celebrated one of their bank holidays, around the time of our Memorial Day. Since all my family's London friends would be away during that time, I had made arrangements to visit Alice and Sister Dee in Devon.

Taking out the garbage the Thursday night before I was to leave, I tripped and fell down three cement steps. When I got up, I felt a sharp pain in my right ankle, but I still managed to make it back to my apartment. The next morning I was in so much pain that it was excruciating for me to move my foot, and I couldn't stand on it. But pain was nothing new to me, so I did what I had to do, got dressed and crawled my way to the phone in the hall, calling NCK to say I wouldn't be coming in. I then phoned Devon and told the sisters what had happened and that I wouldn't be able to visit them.

I knew I should see a doctor, but I didn't know whom to call. For some reason, I decided to phone my friends the Griffins, hoping they were still home and could give me their doctor's name. The phone rang and I was afraid that they might have already left. But I was in luck. Nadia Griffin finally answered. I explained my situation and said I was sorry to phone, knowing that she was probably just leaving for her week away.

"That's all right," she said. "But it's a holiday weekend, so I doubt if most doctors will be around. But stay by the phone, Albert, and I'll call you right back."

Soon the phone rang. "Albert," Nadia said, "I'll be by in about an hour to pick you up and you can sit in our garden and spend the weekend with us. Our doctor is around and he'll see you this afternoon."

Several hours later in the Griffin home, I felt a gentle hand on my shoulder. It was Griff. "Sorry," he said, "you must have been having some good dreams, but it's time for your appointment with our doctor. I hope he'll find it's nothing serious."

Soon we were in the doctor's office. I had thought ahead and brought with me the letter my doctor in America had written concerning the state of my health.

After looking it over and giving me a thorough examination, the doctor told me that I only had a bad sprain and that it should heal with just a few days of rest.

"That's a relief," I said with a sigh. "How much do I owe you?"

"That won't be necessary," the doctor said. "You're a friend of the Griffins and they took care of it."

Over the next three days, with Griff helping me to keep the weight off my foot, my ankle felt better. By Monday I was walking up those three flights of stairs by myself.

During my lunch hour the next day, I found a florist a block away from NCK's office. At about four o'clock that afternoon, the phone at my desk rank. It was Nadia.

"A garden just appeared in my kitchen," she said. "You didn't have to do that."

"Well, it's the least I could do. I just can't get over everything you did for me. And besides, I had such a good time and enjoyed being with you."

For the next five and a half years I saw the Griffins on and off, but I always spent Mother's Day with Nadia, each time sending another "garden" the day before. Her own son and daughter were teenagers, away at boarding school, so I became her adopted son and she became my London mother.

I always looked forward to those Mother's Day Sundays. Griff would pick me up in the morning, deliver me to Nadia and then return me to my apartment that evening after a delicious high tea at their home. Nadia would pack a picnic lunch, but before eating she and I would walk through Kensington Gardens, hand in hand, stopping by the round pond to feed the fish and watch people sail their small boats.

More than thirty years would pass until our paths would cross again. During that time I never forgot the Griffins' kindness. When I pass a florist I remember Nadia's pleasure at the "gardens" I sent her. I wish that I could see them again and tell them that their acts of kindness will never be forgotten. And now I realize that they are not only not forgotten, but also that the memory of our friendship has often served to heal some of the wounds that life keeps on inflicting.

One of these wounds occurred not long ago when I was waiting in a checkout line at a supermarket. A woman in line moved in front of me and put her groceries on the counter. Although I had been standing in line for some time, and my legs had started to become painfully cramped, it seemed too late to say anything because the cashier was already ringing up some of the woman's items. I left with the feeling that both women thought they had "put one over" on that handicapped man. Although it was a trivial incident, for the rest of the day I was filled with angry thoughts about what a mean and rotten world I lived in.

Finally, though, I remembered how in the past I have helped myself to deal with these painful, negative feelings by turning my thoughts to the Griffins. Soon my spirits are lifted and I'm ready to fight another day.

For me, the Griffins' behavior represents one of life's mysteries. What makes some people so giving and others so selfish? I have no answers to this question. I do know, however, that the Griffins came into my life at a time when I needed them most. They reminded me that the world is full of all sorts of people. They reminded me that if you are patient and open to new experiences, you have a good chance of finding people like the Griffins. And they helped me to remember that if you keep these people alive in your heart, they can lead you through life's many dark days and on into the light.

A footnote to the Griffins: I'm happy to say that we're back in contact and are on each other's Christmas card lists. We have also seen each other on my trips to New York City which I still manage to make once a year.

Another interesting person I met was Jean. She was an interior decorator and a good friend of my parents. She helped me set up a real nice apartment at #10B The Drive. The two of us got along so well that we even started dating for a time. She was divorced and I got a kick out of telling people that I was going out with a woman old enough to be my father, as she was three years older than my mother. We had fun going out to dinner and to the theater. She even took me to parties where I got to meet some famous people. I would have another encounter with an older woman. This time she was thirty-six, I was twenty-eight. She would turn out to be a lifelong friend.

During my time in London I got involved in many local civic clubs and organizations. One of these clubs was the music club of London, which combined its activities with wine tastings. We would visit a local winery and would not only taste the wine, but also learn a little bit about the country where the wine came from, i.e., Italy, France and Germany, just to name a few. As you can imagine, the management of the various wineries wanted us to taste their most expensive wines, hoping that we would buy a few bottles.

The group that came to the wine tastings was different from the ones who attended the music events. I did both and got to meet a lot of interesting people by just enjoying what's there.

One of these people was Rosemary. She was older than me but we soon became friends and are still friends today. One evening she stopped me in the hall after a club meeting and asked me if I wanted to stop for coffee before heading home. I said, "Sure, that would be nice," but had a soft drink instead since I don't drink coffee. One thing led to another and I asked her to a concert at the Royal Festival Hall. She said, "That would be wonderful, and maybe we could have dinner at Festival Hall. I have never been there, but I heard it's lovely."

Little did I know I was in for a little romance. The romantic part didn't last simply because I found myself not to be in love with Rosemary, but I'm happy to say that we have remained the best of friends up until this day. And that might be even better than being unhappy lovers.

Dinner at the Festival Hall was indeed lovely. The restaurant looked over the Thames River. Rosemary asked me how much the tickets were and then said that she wanted to pay for dinner because she believed in women's liberation. Since it was the 70s and women's liberation was all the rage, I had no objections and handed over the check with no argument.

Rosemary was also smart. She played three musical instruments and had an ear for language, speaking both French and German. On some days, when we would get together, she would read to me in German.

One of the things I liked about Rosemary was that she never questioned my actions. When I said I had gone to Boston University, she only said, "Good for you!" She never inquired after my major and why I only worked as an information officer for an advertising agency, and later why I only sold publications for a housing organization. It was nice just being able to be oneself and enjoy activities with another person who enjoyed them, too.

Rosemary was married twice. I didn't know the first husband since he had died when Rosemary was only twenty-two. She was still very much attached to him.

I must say here that we had a bit of sex thrown into our relationship. But seeing she was still very much attached to her dead husband and I was still attached to Jackie, we remained just good friends.

Rosemary did end up getting married again, again to an older man. I had moved back to the States by then, but I would stay at their home on my London visits. He was a real nice guy and used to tell me how fond Rosemary was of me and how he was also pleased that I worked and was so involved in the life around me.

Besides the music club, I joined the English Speaking Union where, here again, I met two nice women who became life-long friends, Sue and Rita.

When I moved to #10B The Drive I really started to get involved in community affairs. And that was when I met the Barbours, a lovely older couple. They lived around the corner and would drive me around town. It was through them that I was introduced to the Camden Community Council. The year was 1974 and the United Nations had designated it the Year of Population Control. It ended in a big population conference in Bucharest, Romania, which I luckily attended.

I have been interested in the population problem ever since high school. I had realized that the world was getting too crowded, and with more people, not only was there a loss of freedom, but a scarcity of resources as well.

I also believed that every baby born in the world should be a wanted baby, so there needed to be good access to education about birth control. With these ideas in mind, I was off to the first meeting of the Camden Council in London, which luckily was not too far from where I lived. I arrived by taxi and was taken home by the Barbours.

The group took to me right away and soon I found myself organizing an exhibit incorporating my ideas on population vs. freedom. That was so successful it was used by other groups around town. The UN, in other years, had other conferences. One year, with the Barbours' help, I was able to go to a meeting in Vancouver, Canada.

I was able to join other community groups as a representative of the Camden Council—Friends of the Earth, and the United Nations Association, to name **two**. The council needed to be represented so they were more than happy to have me so willing, and they paid the yearly membership fee. I was spoiled because when I moved back to the States and joined these same groups, I found I was on my own and had to cough up those membership fees. Oh, well, the free ride was fun while it lasted. I also got a free membership in the Music Club of London one year, as I was the only one who took them up on their offer and introduced three people to the group who became members. This gave me a free membership that was good for a year. The management was amazed that somebody actually took them up on their offer. It seems nobody had since the club was founded. And I did it! Who says a disabled man has no friends?

During my years in London I took advantage of my location and managed to take several trips. One of these was to Oslo, Norway. I was on my way to a famous sculpture park, but was afraid I was lost. I stopped a woman on the street and asked her if I was headed in the right direction, and how many more blocks I had to go. To my horror, she told me I was going in the right direction, but that it was ten miles away! Seeing the look on my face, and also noticing that I had trouble walking, she said, "Don't worry. My car is nearby and I'll take you there."

I thanked her profusely, and when we arrived at the park, I offered to pay for the gas and her inconvenience, but she refused saying, "You do something nice for someone else, and it will get back to me."

I've tried many times to do that, and hope that my acts of kindness have somehow gotten back to her.

Besides being helped by that nice woman in Norway, I got a treat when I visited Norway. I was invited to dinner by Norman's managing director. He was American and his pretty blonde wife was Norwegian. They were the nicest people. I learned from them that the Norwegians were very sincere people and only did things out of kindness and really didn't expect favors in return. They don't care if it makes good business sense or not. If a Norwegian was going to feel uncomfortable about his actions, the action wouldn't be done. They were quite interested in my story about the lady who drove me ten miles out of her way and they said they were happy to have met me after all those telexes and letters. I kept in touch for a while, but sadly, we lost contact.

I made many friends over the telex machine and interoffice mailings. I was even able to make arrangements to be met at airports when I went traveling. The people seemed more than happy to help me and it saved me the worry about getting lost or being taken advantage of.

On one of these trips to Denmark I telexed NCK's office in Copenhagen telling them of my dates of arrival and departure and asked if I could be met at the airport. They did just that and billed me for it later when I was safely back in London.

Copenhagen was a fun city. The NCK people put me up in a nice hotel. Yes, besides transportation, they did find me a centrally located hotel. They were also very helpful and organized bus tours for me. I was able to see the city and much of the surrounding countryside with its many castles. I was glad to be walking because I couldn't manage those tour buses today. I could lift my foot higher in those days. Plus, I was steadier on my feet back then. However, I could never walk long distances and usually had to stay in the bus and wait for a report from my fellow travelers. I did go out on my own at night and one night ventured into Copenhagen's Red Light District. The girls did not seem terribly attractive and I was surprisingly left alone. Seeing my condition, I was an easy target for someone. But I did get a kick out of seeing what went on. I also was bold enough to walk right into a building that was staging a live sex show. There was a rough group of men in the audience but again, as soon as they saw me come in they settled down and one of them came over to me and believe it or not, helped me to a seat in the front row and said, in broken English, "Enjoy the show."

"Thanks," I said, as the man left to join his buddies.

The show started and I got a kick out of the fact that the girls stripped along to the music. The music would stop (I guess the place didn't own a tape recorder and they used records that had to be turned over) and they would stop, too, in mid-strip, until the music continued. It was the funniest thing. Again, the girls looked "slutty," so not very attractive. But the evening was an experience none-theless. Till this day, whenever I hear those particular songs, my mind can't help but make the connection to that evening.

When the show was over, I again made my own way. A taxi stopped and drove me back to the hotel. The driver was amazed to see that I was unmolested, seeing that the street I walked down was known to be one of the most dangerous in the city. I guess the whole evening came down to my lifelong philosophy of facing the world without fear.

I did manage to purchase some x-rated books to bring back to friends in England and America.

There were a few more trips, to Yugoslavia and Switzerland. But none would top the time I had in Denmark, even though the others did have their moments, too.

In Yugoslavia I went out on my own and got myself a haircut, but was shocked when I went to pay the man to find that I had no money. "How could I do such a thing as leave my hotel without my wallet? How could I be so stupid?" I said to myself. The man was kind and pointed to the number five on his watch. I had two hours to find my way back to the hotel and return with the money. "I'll be back," I told him and quickly left. Well, as it turned out, I never returned and I bet the man is still cursing Americans till this day. The reason I didn't return was I simply got lost. I wandered the street trying desperately to find my hotel. Finally, I saw a group of soldiers standing behind a fence. "Oh, good," I said to myself. "These soldiers might speak English and steer me in the direction of my hotel." Was I wrong!

They spoke English all right, but instead of directions, one of the men said, "Come with me," and led me into a building that seemed to be the main office. What was going on? I only asked the guy for directions back to my hotel.

Well, I soon found out that I had wandered onto a strategic Russian army base and the secret police wanted to have a word with me.

I should have been scared, but I wasn't. I simply thought that I only had to tell the truth, and all would be well. After all, I wasn't a spy for my Uncle Sam. How-ever, a few action photos with the soldiers in front of those Russian tanks would make valuable souvenirs for the group back home and in London. I decided, however, to be good once I was face-to-face with the head of the camp's secret police. He asked me how I came to be there. I just told him the truth. I was terrible when it came to directions and just got lost and needed to get back to the hotel for dinner. I didn't mention the barber.

After half an hour of telling the police the same story, I was free to leave. I guess I wasn't as big a threat as they thought. A pity, as I was in need of a real adventure to tell the folks back home. Oh well, I guess being at least interrogated by the secret police in a Communist country was adventure enough.

Luckily, the interrogator was kind and sensing my concern had his comrade drive me back to the hotel.

He drove me back in an old Volkswagen. I was just in time for dinner. At dinner I told our guide about the barber and he told me not to worry, barbers are taken care of by the state.

There were other adventures such as when the coal miners went on strike in England. As I remember it they were out for about six weeks. I was living in my apartment in Hampstead and luckily it was close enough to Royal Free Hospital to be connected to their generator, so while the rest of Britain was "dark," I was in the light. I was interested to observe that even though there was no light the crime rate was down.

When I moved again I had to register my new address with the police. I was an alien and had to carry a green card during most of my stay in England. I went to the police station the day of the World Cup finals. The policeman who filled out my papers was good humored, and smiling said, "You would have to bother us with this today, of all days."

I met John Standish through my involvement with Friends of the Earth and Stan worked with me during my years at NCK. I've known John since 1973 when he was living with another woman. With his new wife Jennifer we still manage to get together when I'm in London and e-mail each other often. John is quite the intellectual and a member of Mensa. He has always been impressed at the way I kept my mind alive, always challenging him, and everyone else, to do their best and make a difference.

John also told me that having a mother named Rea (Rhea being the mother of the gods), he wouldn't be surprised about anything I might achieve.

I also have fond memories of the local Unitarian Church. I sold their publications during the weekly service and attended many church events.

As you can see I had a good time and a lot of memories from my England days. I feel very fortunate to have had the experience of living in Europe those many years and that I was physically fit to enjoy my life no matter where it took me.

Now, I was heading back stateside. What new adventures awaited me there? I was just about to turn thirty when my plane landed in Boston that November morning in 1976.

# 4

## *Boston*

◆

### *November 1976–November 1977*

Boston was not the same place I remembered from my college days seven years earlier. Boston is really a college town and I was no longer in college nor was I in the medical field or part of a church or government organization. I was a marketing/publication guy. I almost landed a job in the publication office at MIT. The woman was impressed with my knowledge and background gained at Shelter. But as soon as she heard that I couldn't type, the offer of a job was withdrawn. I thanked her for her efforts and moved on.

To give me something to do, and a place to go in the meantime, I answered an ad placed by an environmental agency that was looking for people to monitor local papers and clip any articles they saw dealing with environmental issues. The articles would then be put into files and used by environmentalists as hard data when they went to lobby various government offices. The office was right next to the statehouse, too. The office of The Friends of the Earth was just down the street. I decided to offer my services there, too. Both these offices were located on Beacon Hill, a very posh area of the city. There were even cobblestone streets, just like some of the streets in London.

Even though I was enjoying the work, it wasn't gaining me a paycheck or the respect of my peers. I was sorry to come to the realization that Boston was great for when I was a student but despite how I tried, it held no future for me now that I was an adult. If I wanted to really "be a part of it all," a move further south to New York would have to be made.

One Sunday a woman I worked with at the environmental clipping service place took me to her church where a fortuneteller was doing a service. It was there that I was told that I was about to move south to New York. I wasn't one to believe in fortunetellers, but I thought what she had to say on the subject was interesting. As she predicted, I ended up spending only one year in Boston.

I knew she was right. My time was running out, better make the most of my remaining time in Boston. I joined a community theater group, which was putting on the musical *Guys and Dolls*. The group was located in a poorer part of the city, namely Roxbury.

Roxbury was well known to me as the place of the bad race riots of the late 1960s and early 70s. Since I hadn't heard anything bad about Roxbury lately, I wasn't that concerned about my safety. I would just have to be very focused and act unafraid.

Mission Hill, the name of the group as well as the section of Roxbury, had a very large membership, mostly working class folks who loved theater. I was welcomed with open arms, and was immediately put in charge of the group's publicity as well as the show's program. The program I came up with included cast bios. This was the first time the group ever tried a program of this magnitude. The show was a big success. But then again, who doesn't like *Guys and Dolls*.

The traveling proved not to be a problem. I went by taxi cab and as the rehearsals progressed one of the women in the group would give me a lift home. As I remember she was kinda cute but alas was already married. Oh, well!

I also became active in the Arlington Street Unitarian Church. This time the place held the same magic for me as it did when I attended services back in my college days. During this stay in Boston the pulpit was manned by one Victor Carpenter. He had spent many years in South Africa, was very thought-provoking and a real social activist. I learned later that one of his children had cerebral palsy.

The church was one of the places I would miss when I finally left Boston.

As for my living quarters in Boston, my parents had found me a one-bedroom apartment in a brand new building. 221 Massachusetts Avenue was built with space for retail stores. There were only a few places already taken. I saw the ice cream parlor that I used to frequent during my college days. It was practically next door to Symphony Hall, the home of the Boston Symphony.

I would meet my friend Dick Prescott there for dinner whenever he was in the area. I had met Dick when he married my friend Gill, who worked with me in London, at NCK. The friendship is still very strong today.

The building also had its own police force that had a regular beat all around the building. I wouldn't get to know these guys well until the spring, when I started to take a wooden folding chair I purchased up to the roof garden to enjoy the evening air. How I was ever able to carry the chair from my ninth floor apartment was anyone's guess. But manage it, I did. And I still have that folding chair today.

I also managed to take a course at Boston University in urban development. My days with Shelter were not wasted and I added much to the class discussion. I hadn't been in a college classroom in eight years and felt right at home. As my father always said, never judge what Albert knows from test scores alone.

A local housing organization also found my volunteer help useful.

I felt that something was missing even though I knew money would never be an issue.

I needed the respect that came with holding down a full-time job.

# 5

## *Scarsdale*

♦

### *November 1977–June 1997*

I delayed leaving Boston as long as I could, even spending the last two days in a local hotel. But alas, no job, so one Friday morning shortly after my thirty-first birthday I boarded a train heading for Stamford, Connecticut where my parents would meet me and drive me the rest of the way to Scarsdale and my new home on Garth Road, #230. Once again my parents came through and found me a great apartment. I thanked them, promising that I hoped to live there for many years and that their apartment hunting days on my behalf were over.

The lobby of 230 was located on the second floor and since my apartment was on the fourth floor I started walking down and up the two flights of stairs. I continued this activity for the next fifteen years until my legs started to give out. I looked forward to the climb as it made me feel that I lived in a two-story house instead of a nine-floor apartment building.

Seeing that my parents left me shortly after arriving at my new home, I wasted no time in exploring my new surroundings.

Garth Road had some lovely Tudor buildings, and I noticed as I walked along that there was a nice restaurant located at the end of my street. I ended up having my dinner there most Saturday evenings before the restaurant closed its doors for good.

Crossing the street I came face to face with C Town, a big supermarket. As soon as I walked in, I noticed the large selection of frozen foods. I knew I would be taking advantage of it soon. My parents had left me with a well-stocked freezer so I didn't have to do any shopping. During my little walk around I ran into the store's manager. He was a nice young man who assured me that his staff would be more than willing to help me when the time came. He welcomed me into the neighborhood.

I walked into Scarsdale National Bank, too. It was next door to C Town. My parents had mentioned that they had opened up a checking account in my name.

The people were very nice and we talked about also opening a savings account.

The Plaza movie theater came next. The cost for a show was still only ninety-nine cents, a real bargain for a first-rate movie. I was very sad to learn recently that the building was torn down to make room for condos.

The local dry cleaner was next. It was run by a nice Polish family. They too were very nice to me over the years. I remember coming in and cashing some of my personal checks. It was during the Metro-North train strike. The bank was closed by the time I returned from work, but the cleaner was open and was happy to help me cash a check or two. They of course did all my laundry, too.

Finally I came to the Scarsdale railroad station. The whole walk took me about twenty minutes, at my pace, which was not bad.

Monday morning I awoke and got myself ready for my first real job in years. My father had secured me a job with United Cerebral Palsy (UCP) in their purchasing department. It wasn't marketing but I would still be looking up information and writing up purchasing orders instead of marking reports. I couldn't wait to start. In those days I was taking the 7:40 express into the city. I would change that routine shortly and be wide awake on the 6:37. At that point I got a ride to the station with the Arnold Bread delivery truck.

The people on the trains were very friendly and I soon made a lot of friends. Towards the end of my working days I arranged for a railroad employee to meet the train with a wheelchair and wheel me out of the station to a waiting cab.

But in 1977 I was still walking. I first started walking to 23rd Street and Lexington Avenue. It was a good walk from Grand Central Station, which was at 42nd Street. I walked, too, to UCP's new location for the fund raising and finance department, only this time I only had to go to 30th and Madison Avenue.

Shortly after my arrival I got myself involved with putting on UCP's annual telethon and worked around the clock.

I was enjoying being part of an organization and learning the ins and outs of the purchasing department. It was also a great feeling to be receiving a paycheck every two weeks. I soon found out that my bank in Scarsdale was open Thursday nights until seven. I arranged to obtain my paycheck a day early so I could take advantage of the Thursday late closing. I deposited it early so I would not misplace my check over the weekend.

I took out a subscription to the local weekly paper, *The Scarsdale Inquirer.* One week I saw an article about a writing class in which the teacher, Louise Albert, believed that everyone had a story to tell. A few months earlier I had written my mother's second cousin, Joan. She had been writing on golf for *Sports Illustrated* for many years and thought since it had been awhile since we were last in communication, it might be fun to bring her up to date on what was happening with the Eliases. I guess it was an entertaining account and well-written because I received an answer back stating that I should start writing more. She said that my funny and informative style would appeal to a reader. It was with this thought in mind that I wrote to Louise Albert explaining what I was writing and did she think she could be of any help?

Well, Louise indeed phoned and we arranged to meet that Saturday around 10:30. Since I couldn't drive we arranged that I would take a taxi to her home and that her husband Floyd would drive me home.

Saturday came and the taxi found the Albert's carriage house on Park Road without much difficulty.

I had brought with me a piece I was working on about Jackie. We wasted no time getting down to work. Louise thought it best that we cover three pages in the one-hour sessions. We met every other Saturday during my years in Scarsdale.

After each session with Louise she would either give me tea and cookies or if she had more time I would stay for lunch. During our talks I learned that her husband had gone to college with my boss Norman Kimball (I always wondered if Mr. Kimball was related to Professor Kimball who helped me out at Boston University those many years ago. I never found out. But there is one thing I do know and that is that both men were very kind to me and looked after my best interests. I'm an independent guy and need an environment that allows me to remain so. During my years with UCP I was known as an independent executive. I have managed to go through life unharmed doing the best I can, thanks in part to people like the Kimballs who didn't let people mess with me.)

With every session with Louise my writing just got better and better. Then one winter's day in 1983 Scarsdale experienced one of its worst snowstorms in years. I had tickets to see a ballet that Saturday afternoon and didn't let the storm, or anything else for that matter, stop me from seeing some pretty fancy footwork.

I managed to not only get myself to the Scarsdale train station but to Lincoln Center as well. The "anything else" turned out to be a mugging, but I was not hurt and carried on.

The ballet, *A Midsummer Night's Dream*, was wonderful.

I wrote about my adventure and Louise helped me submit the piece to the Westchester section of the *New York Times*. They not only printed the article but had it illustrated as well. Needless to say, I was thrilled beyond belief. I also got a little monetary compensation for my efforts. But the best thing of all was my neighbors' reactions. I had people coming up to me for weeks telling me how much they enjoyed reading my piece, even a teacher, who had her students cut it out of the paper and bring it into the classroom so that a discussion could take place. The whole experience was too good to be true.

There would be seven other works published in various papers before my years in Scarsdale would come to a close.

Those first three years of living in Scarsdale were mostly taken up by getting up five days a week, meeting my commuting buddies, going to work and coming home. I took myself out to the local restaurant for a meal on Saturday night before catching a movie. I attended a local Unitarian church on Sundays. I managed to get a ride with some local people. The Elseviers were Dutch and were more than willing to drive me. They were kind enough to have me back to their home afterwards for some lunch and a nip of sherry. They often kidded me, saying if they really needed to say something to each other they would just speak Dutch. I was also included in some theater outings, summer barbeques and being asked to write something that would be part of an anniversary book celebration. I'm still in touch with the Elseviers at Christmas time and never forget their anniversary.

Towards the end of my stay I attended a smaller Unitarian Society and got involved in writing and doing a few of their programs. *Doing the Best I Can* was one I did about what Unitarianism meant to me. Another I remember was *All About Kindness*. I'm still somewhat involved with this society today and in touch at Christmas and through e-mail with many of its members: Stu & Barbara Caplan, Bill Holstein, Gil & Bonnie Hart, Lisa DeMauro and Walter & Doris Staubi, among others.

Besides church activities I was destined to add a lot of new activities to my life as well.

One of these was community theater, shades of Boston.

I was reading the *Scarsdale Inquirer*, as was my Friday night habit. The police reports were especially entertaining. If any of these complaints happened in other parts of New York, they would seem so trivial that the police would be laughing their heads off. I guess that is one of the reasons people who choose to live in the area feel it is very safe. Anyway, after reading the police reports I saw an article about Greenville Community Theatre. The president, Peter Tea, was asking for new members. I contacted him and arrangements were made to attend the next meeting of the group.

I enjoyed my time at the meeting, and over the years made many close friends: the Korsens, Blooms, Herberts, Teas, Goldbergs, Specter, Forstenzers and Boylans, to name a few.

The group held monthly meetings and put on small one-act productions and two full-length plays annually, plus had many cast parties. After I had attended the group's events for a couple of years, Tony Herbert asked me if I would like to help him publicize the group's monthly workshops.

I was delighted, as I loved writing. They must have liked what I did as I was asked to remain in my position for the remainder of my time with the group.

Peter Tea also contacted me about being in a workshop with Bern. I was remembering my one and only acting experience. It was 1961 and I was asked to do a scene from Shakespeare's *Macbeth*. My performance in class was good enough to perform in front of the whole school. Could I do it again?

I told Peter, yes, I could do it. The next evening he was at my front door with a copy of Eugene O'Neill's *Hughie*. I took the copy from Peter and started leafing through the pages. I immediately noticed that my character, that of the night clerk, is seated behind a desk during the whole show so I wouldn't have any problems with moving around the stage or with standing. The only movement comes at the very end of the play, and Bern would help me.

Here I leave the theater group for a moment to mention that the Scarsdale Inquirer also played a role in connecting me with the local Audubon Society. The president took me to the first meeting and immediately asked me to join the board of directors and become their publicity chairman. I was very keen about communing with nature, so why not take him up on his offer. Besides the Schoenfelds, I became friends with Martha Creamer, the Frankels, Spiros and Elizabeth Stecker.

Back to the theater group. I decided to give the workshop my best shot.

Peter was delighted. My part, that of a night clerk in a small New York hotel in the mid 1920s, made me think of days gone by. Were people less in a hurry living simpler lives? They surely weren't all like Erie Smith, played by Bern, a wise guy and small-time gambler who was part of the rackets. I guess humans have always been a mixture of the good and bad. For Erie Smith had some sentimental softness to him.

The night clerk was a real loner who showed no emotion of any kind. I'm alone, too, but my inner life makes sure that I'm really never alone.

The audience loved the performance, even my adding of a Cole Porter song in the beginning, "Love for Sale." We were even invited to stage performances in front of two local nursing homes. Here, too, we were a hit. For the age of our audience, a lot of the names mentioned in the play, such as Arnold Rothstein, brought back many memories of the period.

As time went by I got my chance to act again, this time in a major fall show, *Twelve Angry Men*. I had a bit part, the judge. My off-stage voice charged the jury as the play opened. I did it live and really felt I was part of the show.

Again, I thank Tony Herbert and the director Rick Cortellessa for giving me yet another opportunity to act.

Scarsdale commuting had its funny side, too. One morning as I was making my way to the train station, a car pulled up beside me and the passenger side door opened. Normally when this happened the driver would ask me if I would like a lift somewhere. This time, however, nothing was said so I just got in the car. The woman behind the wheel then asked, "Are you going to the train station?" I said yes, and then noticed that the back door was starting to open and a man was getting into the backseat. I then realized that the door wasn't being opened for me but for him. We all had a good laugh and headed off to catch the train into New York City. They were great sports and whenever we would run into each other in Scarsdale Village they would always ask if I needed their help.

I met many interesting people on my walks and miss that part of my life now that I can't walk that far. I met ladies of the evening, too, only it was seven in the morning so they were just getting off "work." Glad I was a part of it all for some many years.

There was one great act of kindness given to me by another Peter, the Arnold Bakery truck driver who drove me from my home to the station four days a week.

It happened one snowy day and I was grateful for the help even though snow is a sort of metaphor for me, since it's a challenge but it does not stop me. I traveled in it for many years. Snow didn't stop me nor for that matter does anything else.

It was Peter who phoned my parents to give them the news that I was having trouble walking and that my stay in Scarsdale was almost at an end. I was able to hold out another year.

I will never forget Peter's kindness. I also remember one Christmas. I had given him a present for his kindness. He looked at me and said, "It should be me who is giving the present. Just seeing your smiling face every morning is a gift in itself. You do much more for me than I bet I have ever done for you."

My time with Peter remains a mystery. Why are some people so giving and others not?

Another mystery person who came in to my life is Marion. It was on a Friday, late afternoon, when I first met Elien Whiting, Marion's mother. I had just gotten a notice from the post office that a package was waiting for me there. Elien said that if I was downstairs the next morning at around nine that they would be more than happy to drive me to pick it up. I was and they did. What I thought was a single trip turned out to be a Saturday morning event: post office, shoe repair, grocery shopping, cleaners and a lift to Louise Albert's every other Saturday, not to mention wine bottle openings and fish feeding when I was away. I guess I forgot to mention that I have fish tanks, two at the moment.

All during this period I never stopped going to concerts and plays. In the mid 1980s I met a new friend while waiting for the train.

Lorraine Miller was a tall redhead and we immediately struck up a conversation. One thing led to another, and before I knew it I had asked her out to the theater and to my amazement she said yes. Till that moment I had either gone by myself or with Jane Goldberg, a gal I had met during my years at Boston University. We remain good friends to this day. Jane stopped off in London to spend a few days with me on her way back from Israel and accompanies me to theater and the ballet whenever she's available. She was very instrumental in introducing me to my friend Susan. More about Susan later.

For now, it's Lorraine's turn. It was time for the New York City Ballet's annual fall gala. I decided to ask Lorraine and to my delight she again said yes.

As the evening ended and it was time to leave Lincoln Center, the weather took a turn for the worst. A sleet and hale storm had started. I hoped we could make it to the car I hired in one piece. I didn't want Lorraine to ruin her new dress. Lorraine right at that moment sprang into action, turning herself into a "Scarsdale bag lady," even producing a small umbrella to keep us both dry.

That was just one of many adventures we had. The New York City Ballet played a part in a more personal way as well. I was starting to have problems with my right knee, finding it very hard to stand or walk. Lorraine again reached into her bag of tricks, only this time coming out with a quarter, and said, "Stay here while I make a phone call." When she came back a few minutes later, she helped me to the main entrance of the hall and her friend's car that she had arranged to take us both home. I'm happy to say that Lorraine's friendship, too, has stood the test of time and to this day despite the distance we manage to stay in touch by phone and e-mail.

Another place I frequented with Lorraine or just by myself was the Carlyle Hotel and the Café Carlyle. I sometimes spent a weekend in New York, staying at the Carlyle, taking in a Broadway show and hearing Bobby Short doing his cabaret act. It was only once a year so I felt I had a right to treat myself to an early Christmas gift. And besides, the staff of the hotel was just so wonderful and helpful to me. They made me feel I was home. They couldn't have been nicer. Everyone was so helpful making me feel part of the family. I'm truly grateful to have had the experience.

Going to the Café Carlyle brought into focus the great love I have of the American songbook. I have mentioned before how music is a big part of my life and helps my imagination become very creative. My earliest memories of hearing this style of music is when my grandparents took me to hear Billy Eckstine sing when I was only twelve years old. The year was 1959 and from that moment on I was hooked on the music of the 30s and 40s. Some twenty years later I heard my second live performance. This time it was Hugh Shannon. I really enjoyed hearing that "Saloon Singer." I learned that he died shortly afterwards.

That was followed up with an evening of George Gershwin; this time the music was song by Mr. Michael Feinstein. I remember that I got sick on the food but loved the music.

I wanted to hear more, but where could I go? Then in 1989 I got my answer. It came in the form of an invitation to attend the first cabaret convention hosted by the Mabel Mercer Foundation and a Mr. Donald Smith. The evening would consist of the music of Cole Porter and be held at Town Hall in New York City. The only catch was the cost. I almost passed out when I saw how much a ticket cost. I immediately sat down and wrote to Donald Smith, explaining my situation and how much I loved the music of Mr. Cole Porter. To my amazement, a week later I got a note from Mr. Smith, thanking me for my interest and little donation (since I could not afford the ticket, I sent what I could) and said, "Enjoy the evening. We took care of you." I certainly did enjoy myself and have attended the convention many times now that the prices are more reasonable.

I was very happy to see that the convention provides handicap seats now so that others with my condition can enjoy this type of music, too.

My tastes in music really didn't stop with Cabaret. They extended to classical as well. I remembered my days in London with Rosemary and decided to continue the pleasure in New York by attending the ballet and concerts at both Carnegie Hall and Lincoln Center. Here, too, I took a friend I met at Cerebral Palsy, Mary Ann Carroll. We are still in contact by e-mail today.

Time went by, then one night my friend Jane, whom I stayed in contact with from my days at Boston University, had me over for dinner. During the dinner Jane got an unexpected phone call from her neighbor, Susan Horowitz. Jane informed Susan that she was entertaining an old friend from college but that Susan was free to stop by for dessert.

Susan indeed stopped by, and on first seeing her something told me that we would be seeing a lot of each other in the future.

Jane noticed, too, that I was becoming interested and said, "Do you want her phone number?" After a moment or two of just staring into Susan's eyes, I said, "Yes, I would."

Susan reached into her purse and handed me her business card.

On the way home I wondered if we would really ever meet again. I noticed an ad in the *New York Times* that the New York City Ballet would be performing Friday of the following week. I asked Susan if she would like to attend the performance.

Asking Susan out proved to be a performance in itself. It was a written note that sealed the match.

I received my answer shortly. The phone rang a little after 8 P.M. The voice on the other end of the line said, "Albert Elias? This is Susan Horowitz. I got your note asking me out to the ballet. It was a very lovely letter, taking me by surprise as I have never been asked out this way before, by letter I mean. I've given your offer a lot of thought and yes, let's go."

A date with a stranger, someone other than Jane or Lorraine, how nice.

It would prove to be a rough ride for the first couple of years until our feelings for each other were sorted out. Susan and I have become best friends and in some cases our relationship has become closer than most marriages. And even though we don't have a physical relationship, it's more than compensated for by the joy of life and for the arts that we both share and the happiness we both feel just being in each other's company.

Jackie will forever be my soul mate and live in my imagination. And now I have Susan's company to share the activities we both love. One can't ask for more.

In 1997 I left Scarsdale and moved to Florida. I was starting to have real health problems.

I'll miss my life at Cerebral Palsy and the challenges and encounters I had just getting there. My bosses, a Mr. Tim Whooley and Mr. Dan Capone, were very friendly and helpful. I'm happy that we all stayed in touch via phone, e-mail and Christmas cards.

During the summer of 1996 I had an MRI done on my right knee but it showed nothing. I rested it that whole summer and just read and listened to books on tape. I was fighting hard to hang in there.

I knew I would really never leave New York, for a big part of me would remain. My spirit would go on having various adventures.

In June of 1997 I left Scarsdale for good. A week before my scheduled leaving date of June 16, 1997, I had the most excruciating stomach pain ever. I phone 911 and was rushed to the hospital where it was discovered that I needed to have my gallbladder removed. I decided to remain in the hospital until the 16$^{th}$ and have my gallbladder removed in Florida. My doctor, John Moses, took good care of me those few days. It seemed that we saw more of each other then than we did during my whole twenty years in Scarsdale. We are still in touch at holiday time and now that he is retired and has become a writer himself, I was happy to hear that he has not forgotten me and has included me in his book and poetry.

# 6

## *The Present*

◆

### *June 1997–*

Nine years have passed since I left Scarsdale. My gallbladder has been removed and I suffered a stroke.

Against the advice of my doctors and educators my parents sent me to school when I couldn't walk. I went on to high school both in this country and abroad. My senior year at Greenwich High School was hard at first but I stayed the course. During that year I made many lifetime friends: Lynn, Linda, Fran and Randy all have been wonderful about keeping in touch. Lynn has been especially kind by having me to her homes in Colorado and Kentucky. I have spent Christmas and numerous vacations with her and her family. We also exchange Christmas and birthday gifts along with e-mails and snail mail.

I went on to survive the cold winters of Boston and not only had an education but gained the skills I needed for independent living. Those skills came in handy when I returned to both England and Boston later in life.

In Scarsdale, the window into New York, I used these skills again and played and worked in the area for twenty years.

John Beyersdorf helped me onto the commuter train and also made sure that I got safely through Grand Central Station. We are still in touch today. To him and my many other nameless helpers, I thank you.

In Scarsdale I was also given the chance to act and was part of community theater, and helped save the environment by being a part of the local Audubon Society.

The Westchester Unitarian Society gave me the opportunity to explore my inner self. The Unitarian emphasis on the power of the individual has helped me build a strong inner life and find happiness in doing the best I can.

I was grateful for those fifty years of independence and for the people who helped me by just being made aware of their own humanity. I was told by a taxi driver who helped me one day that he was first a human being, then a taxi driver. We all need help now and then. People would help me and then others seeing from example were not afraid to help, too.

Perhaps it was only fitting to have ended my days in Scarsdale lying in a hospital bed. It made the transition from an independent to an interdependent person less emotional and painful.

After my stroke the doctors weren't too optimistic about my chances. Thanks in part to my nurse and friend, Leneve, and my therapist, Patrick, I was able to make a full recovery.

I'm thankful that my mind has remained intact. Having overcome a stroke has given me a new burst of energy.

I find every day a growing experience and celebrate the mysteries of life all around me.

Jackie is still in my thoughts. Our fantasy dates help keep her alive in my heart. She will remain my soul mate until the day I die. I remain forever thankful for having had the experience.

I'm very grateful for having Susan in my life. We talk on the phone, share our writings, go to theater and share the excitement of visiting places both in the U.S.A. and abroad. I still can make it up to New York and Susan travels to Florida when she can.

I'm grateful for having an understanding family that allowed me to experience life to the fullest. They made it possible for me to develop an inner life and show people that I meet how we both can enjoy a life with more ups than downs.

978-0-595-37213-3
0-595-37213-9

www.ingramcontent.com/pod-product-compliance
Lightning Source LLC
Chambersburg PA
CBHW051447280526
45785CB00003B/1464